D1194833

Community
Pharmacy
Handbook

Community Pharmacy Handbook

Jon Waterfield

BPharm, MSc, MRPharmS, PGCE
Senior Lecturer in Pharmacy Practice and Clinical Pharmacy
Leicester School of Pharmacy, De Montfort University
Leicester, UK

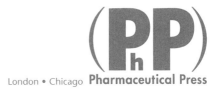

London • Chicago **Pharmaceutical Press**

Published by the Pharmaceutical Press
An imprint of RPS Publishing

1 Lambeth High Street, London SE1 7JN, UK
100 South Atkinson Road, Suite 200, Grayslake, IL 60030-7820, USA

© Pharmaceutical Press 2008

(**PP**) is a trade mark of RPS Publishing
RPS Publishing is the publishing organisation
of the Royal Pharmaceutical Society of Great Britain

First published 2008

Typeset by Photoprint, Torquay, Devon
Printed in Great Britain by TJ International, Padstow, Cornwall

ISBN 978 0 85369 716 9

A catalogue record for this book is available from the British Library

Contents

Preface

With the introduction of the new contractual framework for community pharmacy there are many opportunities for pharmacists to engage in new ways of working. For the community pharmacist this new challenge is both exciting and daunting: exciting in that the pharmacist has many more opportunities to apply their skills as a primary healthcare professional; daunting, as for many pharmacists this is completely new territory. A theme that runs throughout this book is continuing professional development (CPD) and how this essential process can be applied to develop confidence and expertise in new areas of practice. The aim of this book is to provide a spectrum of relevant and accessible information on contemporary community pharmacy practice.

Chapters 1 to 3 are on CPD, applying management skills to community pharmacy and the training and development of the pharmacy team. These introductory chapters recognise that in order to successfully participate in new opportunities, the pharmacist needs to be confident about managing their own development and in turn the training and development of their support team. It is clear that the successful introduction of new services is dependent on the effective management of the whole pharmacy team.

Chapters 4 to 6 include information on the new contractual framework, offering advanced services and the practical issues associated with the delivery of the most popular enhanced services. While much of the content of these chapters relates specifically to the contractual framework in England, many of the practical issues discussed also relate to other national contracts.

Chapters 7 to 9 are on supplying medication, responding to symptoms and multidisciplinary working. These chapters aim to provide an insight into some of the newer ways of working both within the pharmacy and with other healthcare professionals.

The book is designed to answer practical questions such as:

- how do I manage my own professional development?
- what is the best way of motivating and supporting my pharmacy support team?

- what are the practical issues involved in setting up new services?
- how do I work effectively with the primary care team?
- how do I promote the value of pharmacy services?

Clearly this is a challenging and defining time for community pharmacy. Community pharmacists are highly accessible healthcare professionals with many conflicting demands on their time. The overall aim of the *Community Pharmacy Handbook* is to provide a stimulus to encourage new ways of working that will result in increased pharmaceutical care in the community. If this aim is even partially achieved, the effort has been well worth while.

Jon Waterfield
December 2007

How to use this book

In addition to offering support for the community pharmacist, this hand-book will also address some of the learning needs of pharmacy under-graduates and preregistration graduates.

Key features of each chapter

Checkpoint

At the beginning of each chapter there is a short 'Checkpoint' section with some questions to encourage personal reflection on the subject. It is a useful exercise to think about each question before starting to read the chapter.

Implications for practice

At the end of each chapter there are two suggested activities to apply what has been discussed in practice. The activities are only intended as suggested starting points and may lead to other continuing professional development activity.

References and further information

At the end of each chapter a reference and further information section is provided to supplement the text. Many of the references to original doc-umentation have a URL reference. All of the sites have been checked for accuracy and relevance.

Multiple choice questions

There is a set of ten multiple choice questions that relate to each chapter. These questions are designed to mainly test factual recall and provide the opportunity for self-assessment of different subject areas. The questions are written in the style of the Royal Pharmaceutical Society of Great Britain registration examination.

Case studies

An integral part of this handbook is the inclusion of case studies to consolidate the issues and apply the knowledge explored in each chapter. The exercises are aimed at three different levels:

- *level 1*: pharmacy undergraduate student
- *level 2*: preregistration graduate
- *level 3*: community pharmacist.

A set of brief suggested answers for all case studies is provided at the end of the book. The answers are *not* intended to provide a definitive model answer, but to support the reader in the reflection and learning process.

Acknowledgements

I would like to express my sincere thanks to Sandra Hall, Head of Pharmacy Practice, Leicester School of Pharmacy, for reading the manuscript and offering helpful comments and suggestions.

The book would not have been written without the support of my family. Many thanks especially to Alison who encouraged me to embark on this project. Daniel, Anna and Mark ensured that the book was on schedule by regularly asking how many words had been written!

About the author

Jon Waterfield registered as a pharmacist in 1984, having completed his degree at the University of Bradford. Jon qualified as a science teacher and completed his Postgraduate Certificate in Education at the University of Leicester. The early part of his career included teaching science in secondary and further education, both abroad and in the UK. Jon also developed a career within community pharmacy and held various positions as a community pharmacist-manager. In 1993 he completed a pharmaceutical industry research project that resulted in an MSc degree in pharmacology. For several years Jon was national Pharmacy Training Manager for Gehe UK. In 2005 he was appointed Senior Lecturer in Pharmacy Practice and Clinical Pharmacy at Leicester School of Pharmacy, De Montfort University.

Abbreviations

ACE	angiotensin-converting enzyme
ACT	accredited checking technician
AMS	acute medication service
BMI	body mass index
BNF	*British National Formulary*
CD	controlled drug
CE	continuing education
CHD	coronary heart disease
CMP	clinical management plan
CMS	chronic medication service
CPD	continuing professional development
CPMMP	Community Pharmacy Medicines Management Project
CPPE	Centre for Pharmacy Postgraduate Education
CRC	child-resistant container
CSCI	Commission for Social Care Inspection
DDA	Disability Discrimination Act 1995
DOTS	directly observed therapy scheme
DQ	direct questioning
EEA	European Economic Area
ETP	electronic transmission of prescriptions
FH	family history
GMS	general medical services
GP	general practitioner
GSL	general sales list
HbA_{1c}	haemoglobin A_{1c}
HEI	higher education institution
HPC	history of presenting complaint
ICAS	Independent Complaints Advocacy Service
IT	information technology
LPC	local pharmaceutical committee
MAR	medicines administration record
MAS	minor ailment service
MCA	medicine counter assistant

MEP	RPSGB *Medicines, Ethics and Practice* guide
MUR	medicines use review
NatPaCT	National Primary and Care Trust Development Programme
NICE	National Institute for Health and Clinical Excellence
NPA	National Pharmacy Association
NPSA	National Patient Safety Agency
NRT	nicotine-replacement therapy
NSAID	non-steroidal anti-inflammatory drug
NSF	National Service Framework
NVQ	National Vocational Qualification
OTC	over-the-counter
P	pharmacy medicine
PC	presenting complaint
PCC	primary care contracting
PCO	primary care organisation
PCT	primary care trust
PDP	personal development plan
PGD	patient group direction
PHS	public health service
PI	prescription intervention
PIL	patient information leaflet
PMH	past medical history
PMR	patient medication record
PNA	pharmaceutical needs assessment
POM	prescription only medicine
PPD	Prescription Pricing Division
PSNC	Pharmaceutical Services Negotiating Committee
QOF	Quality and Outcomes Framework
RCA	root cause analysis
RPSGB	Royal Pharmaceutical Society of Great Britain
SH	social history
SLA	service level agreement
SMART	specific, measurable, achievable, relevant and timed
SOP	standard operating procedure
SSRI	selective serotonin reuptake inhibitor
SVQ	Scottish Vocational Qualification
SWOT	strengths, weaknesses, opportunities, threats
TNA	training needs analysis
WCPPE	Welsh Centre for Pharmacy Postgraduate Education
WML	Waste Management Licensing (Regulations)

Continuing professional development

Twenty years from now you will be more disappointed by the things you didn't do than by the ones you did do. So throw off the bowlines. Sail away from the safe harbour. Catch the trade winds in your sails. Explore. Dream. Discover.

(Mark Twain)

Checkpoint

Before reading on, think about the following questions to identify your own knowledge gaps in this area:

- What are some of the issues that resulted in the introduction of a formalised approach to continuing professional development (CPD) for healthcare professionals?
- How do you define CPD?
- What is the difference between CPD and continuing education (CE)?
- What is a personal development plan (PDP)?

Continuing professional development (CPD) for the healthcare professional is a theme that runs throughout this book. There are many definitions of CPD and often much confusion about what CPD means in practice. One very simple definition of CPD is: 'everything that you learn that makes you better able to do your job'. The primary aim of the CPD process is to improve the quality of the services we provide as a community pharmacist. The quality of pharmaceutical service provision is increasingly measured by both the public and our paymasters. CPD offers the pharmacist the opportunity to stand back and look at ways of improving their level of professional competence. The fact that you are reading this *Community Pharmacy Handbook* is evidence that you are interested in CPD and developing the way that you practise in the community.

This introductory chapter looks at:

- the origins and drivers for CPD
- the issue of continuously improving quality and clinical governance

- practical issues surrounding CPD and overall personal development planning.

The CPD concept

It is useful at the outset to look at how CPD has come to the forefront of our thinking as a profession and why it is so important. Pharmacy is a respected profession and the community pharmacist is placed in a position of trust, especially in the way that they relate directly to patients and are readily accessible to provide advice and information. CPD involves establishing a framework to ensure that professional competence is maintained and the public is reassured about the high quality of pharmacy services offered.

The high-profile tragic events at the Bristol Royal Infirmary moved the spotlight on to the competence of healthcare professions. One of the many recommendations from the Bristol Royal Infirmary Inquiry (the Kennedy report) was that it must be part of all healthcare professionals' contracts that they undergo appraisal, CPD and revalidation to ensure that all healthcare professionals remain competent to do their job.[1] The government made it clear that health professions should set up systems of mandatory CPD. CPD for health professionals was also emphasised in *The NHS Plan*,[2] and specifically for pharmacists in *Pharmacy in the Future – Implementing the NHS Plan*.[3,4]

CPD is not only driven by government documentation, it has also become a practical reality due to the rapid increase in knowledge relevant to the practice of pharmacy. The extended role of the community pharmacist that has incorporated a much more clinical emphasis has presented the profession with a challenge. The challenge is to ensure that pharmacists are not only up to date with their pharmaceutical knowledge, but are also fit to practise in terms of skill and application of their knowledge. In the past the emphasis has been on continuing education (CE) and this has taken the form of evening meetings, study days and distance learning. This is not an uncommon approach and CE activities were found in other professions such as medicine, nursing, engineering and law. CPD now replaces the earlier requirement of the Royal Pharmaceutical Society (RPSGB), for all pharmacists to complete 30 hours of CE every year. One of the principles of the *Code of Ethics for Pharmacists and Pharmacy Technicians* is to develop professional knowledge and competence.[5] This will require the pharmacist to undertake and maintain up-to-date evidence of CPD relevant to their field of practice (Principle 5.4). Some pharmacists have difficulty with the CPD concept as they feel more comfortable with a knowledge-based CE approach where they attend a learning event or read a chapter in a text book. The acquisition and updating of knowledge in this way is an important activity and one that is a part of the CPD process. However, it is important that a distinction is made between CE and CPD. After many years of using the CE approach it has become clear that this approach has several disadvantages in terms of ensuring 'fitness for practice'. Some of the problems encountered with CE are:

■ CE events do not include the many day-to-day practice-related activities where significant learning takes place, for example interaction with a colleague or tutorial involvement with a pregistration trainee
■ CE events tend to be passive in their approach and to bypass other ways of learning such as job shadowing another healthcare professional or discussing a case with a general practitioner (GP)
■ CE is not specific for individual pharmacists and their development needs at the time. For example a training evening on a specific topic may not be relevant to the development needs and practice priorities of an individual. The aims and objectives of CE courses and training packages are generally set by the course provider
■ the CE assessment process tends to assess only the knowledge gained as opposed to the impact of that knowledge on the pharmacist's practice.

CE certainly has an important place in our ongoing development, but needs to be incorporated into the wider CPD framework. There are many definitions of CPD as it applies to different professions. One example from the Institution of Civil Engineers is:

> The systematic maintenance, improvement and broadening of knowledge and skills and the development of personal qualities necessary for the execution of professional and technical duties throughout your working life.[6]

There are many similar definitions, and all have common keywords that emphasise the continual ongoing nature of the CPD process, the reference to knowledge, skills and behaviour, and the linking of these to professional practice.

The CPD concept is all about the individual driving their own professional development. To engage fully as a community pharmacist within a changing environment, a positive approach towards CPD is essential. An open approach is needed that allows the pharmacist to stand back and ask questions such as:

■ what service do I want to deliver?
■ what are my development needs in this area?
■ how do I meet these needs?
■ how will I reflect on my development in this area and ensure that the service I offer is of the highest quality?

CPD and clinical governance

Clinical governance has been defined as:

> A framework through which NHS organisations are accountable for continuously improving quality of their services and safeguarding high standards of care by creating an environment in which excellence in clinical care can flourish.[7]

At first sight this formal definition can appear quite complex. Clinical governance is all about how to improve quality. The quality-improvement agenda within the NHS includes setting standards from the National Institute for Health and Clinical Excellence (NICE) and national service frameworks (NSFs) and the monitoring of standards by the Healthcare Commission and others. It is important to recognise that the clinical governance umbrella covers a wide range of activities and processes for improving quality and ensuring professional accountability. These processes include the following areas:

- evidence-based practice
- CPD
- audit
- risk management
- remedying poor performance
- monitoring clinical care
- patient and public involvement
- staff management
- being accountable.

CPD is seen as a fundamental component of the quality-improvement agenda and good professional practice. CPD needs to be directed at areas of practice where enhancement of capability is required.[8] Capability in this case can be defined as the extent to which individuals can adapt to change, generate new knowledge and continue to improve their performance.

The pharmacist is required to recognise the limits of their professional competence, practise only in those areas in which they are competent to do so and refer to others where necessary. This principle of the Code of Ethics is of particular relevance to the community pharmacist who is faced with adapting to new expectations, in terms of services offered and new ways of working.

There is currently wide-ranging discussion about the revalidation of pharmacists and how this may operate in the future. CPD is seen to be an essential component of a much wider revalidation process. For example, a revalidation system may involve some form of practice requirement such as a performance appraisal or a practice audit.

Many community pharmacists, while recognising the importance of CPD, can feel uncertain about where to start in terms of their own professional practice.

CPD – getting started

It is important to get started with the CPD process. Many pharmacists are not engaging fully in CPD and need further support to enable them to do so.[9] The aim of this section is to provide the information and guidance necessary to start the process and incorporate CPD as part of everyday working practice.

Some of the major barriers to CPD that could possibly prevent pharmacists from participating fully in the CPD process are:

- a perception that CPD is time consuming
- a misunderstanding of the CPD process and what is involved for the pharmacist
- difficulties in identifying learning needs and evaluating CPD activities.

With the introduction of mandatory CPD it is imperative that these barriers are broken down to enable practising pharmacists to move towards a more focused approach in their own development. CPD need not necessarily be time consuming. For example, a brief question from a patient regarding their medication may lead the pharmacist to reflect on their current knowledge of a particular drug. This may result in only a small amount of research such as looking at reference sources and later applying this knowledge to the next similar patient query. The first part of this process may only take a matter of minutes. Conversely, if as part of a personal and business development plan a pharmacist decides to become involved in the provision of a smoking-cessation clinic, this will clearly involve a much more detailed approach to the planning and development of knowledge and skills before being able to apply this to practice. Both examples of CPD will take vastly different amounts of time and input. Many pharmacists are already involved in CPD on a daily basis but are failing to plan and record their activity. It is only through the disciplined planning and recording of CPD activities that the pharmacist can obtain a more accurate picture of the amount of time it is taking. It is unfair to say that CPD is time consuming, as much of what constitutes CPD activity is integrated into everyday practice. The practicalities of the planning and recording procedures will be discussed later in this section.

The second barrier is a misunderstanding of the CPD process and what this involves. For example, not all pharmacists understand the difference between CE and CPD, and there are definite differences in pharmacists' attitudes and perceptions of the CPD process.[10] This is not an easy barrier to overcome as it often involves a change in behaviour and working patterns. For example, the community pharmacist who has recently attended a training evening on asthma may file the course material and do nothing further with the information they have gained. Alternatively the pharmacist may return from the same CE event and contact the local asthma nurse to informally discuss one of the case studies on the use of corticosteroids in acute asthma. During the conversation the details of the case become reinforced and the pharmacist arranges a more formal meeting with the asthma nurse to look at ways of working together more closely. It is this latter approach that allows the pharmacist to gather momentum in terms of both individual development and delivering improved patient outcomes.

The third barrier of finding difficulty in identifying learning needs and evaluating CPD activities can only be overcome with increased experience. The identification and driving of our personal learning agenda and development plan is a concept that is relatively new for the community pharmacist. The subsequent evaluation of our CPD is a skill that can only be developed over a period of time. The pharmacist should continually make CPD records and examine what they do with a positive but critical eye. This is one of the reasons why it is so important to get started!

CPD is an ongoing cyclical process of reflection on practice, planning, action and evaluation or reflection on learning (Figure 1.1). It is useful to look at each of these stages in turn.

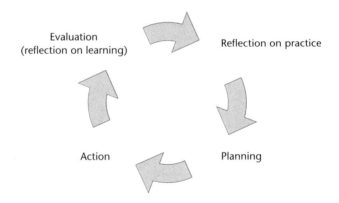

Figure 1.1 The continuing professional development cycle.

Reflection on practice

Reflection on practice is the process that is used to 'self-diagnose' our learning needs. This process involves standing back and looking at what has been achieved in our practice and where we see our career progressing in the future. On a broader scale this is what takes place when

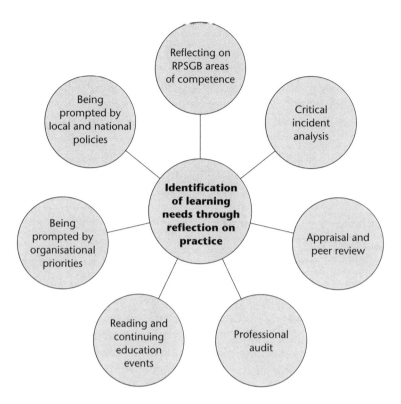

Figure 1.2 Continuing professional development: methods of identifying learning needs through reflection on practice.

we start to write a personal development plan (PDP). It is important to recognise that there are different ways of identifying learning needs through reflection (Figure 1.2). A practical example is included under each heading to illustrate different methods of identifying and highlighting professional development needs.

Examples

All of the examples in this section involve the community pharmacist James Brown, who works for a small multiple in a town centre pharmacy. He has been registered as a pharmacist for 11 years and has worked mainly as a community pharmacist-manager throughout this time.

Critical incident analysis

Critical incident analysis is about learning from meaningful events, and involves taking a thoughtful approach to a particular event and looking at the outcome. It is not important if the outcome to the event was positive or negative. The important issue is that the event is analysed and the question asked: 'What did I do to bring about this positive/negative outcome?'

If the outcome was positive then we are looking at ways of applying our success to other similar situations. If the outcome was negative then we are looking at ways of avoiding a similar situation in the future.

Example 1.1

A customer asks James for his professional opinion on the benefits of taking glucosamine tablets for pain in his knee joint, as he has been recommended to take this by his GP. The customer notes that the product is quite expensive and would like some more information and advice before making the purchase. Glucosamine is not James's specialist subject and he has not read round the subject even though he has been aware of recently published articles on this product. He decides to actively recommend the product as it has been suggested by the GP but finds himself unable to provide an adequate answer to the customer.

On analysis of this incident James feels that he has been put on the spot and not really addressed the query in a professional manner. He starts to think about what his learning needs are in this area and he comes up with two suggestions:

- the need to become more familiar with the use of this product and look critically at the evidence base for its use
- the need to adopt a standard procedure when asked about areas where he has little or no knowledge, for example recording the query and customer details and researching thoroughly before answering the question.

These broad suggestions have stemmed from a critical incident that probably took less than five minutes of James's working day.

Appraisal and peer review

Appraisal and peer review are an excellent way of assessing learning needs. Typically the way we view our own work is often different from the way that our line manager or colleagues see us. For example we may be over-critical of what we do or may have blind spots and areas of development that we tend to ignore. Appraisal tends to be a formal process compared to peer review, which could include an informal conversation. In some cases it is useful to ask a colleague to discuss a critical incident that you are considering, as they may be able to look at the incident from a completely different angle.

Example 1.2

James Brown was talking to his pharmacist friend Ruth Owen about the glucosamine query incident and admitted that he felt that the quality of professional service that he had offered had been less than satisfactory. Ruth mentioned that recently she had experienced a similar incident and this prompted her to contact the medical information department of the glucosamine manufacturer. Ruth obtained some useful reference sources and made some brief notes. Ruth showed James her notes and he was impressed with the way that the papers had been neatly summarised and filed. Ruth suggested that a more organised approach to customer queries and the creation of an accessible file would be useful. Ruth offered to share and explain her system of note taking and filing. This conversation added a new dimension to James's critical incident analysis and identified a further learning need.

Professional audit

A professional audit involves systematic evaluation of professional work against set standards. The process of audit will be discussed in more detail in Chapter 4. Professional audit is a useful tool when reflecting on our learning needs.

Example 1.3

James has noticed recently that a lot of customers have complained about the length of time they need to wait for a prescription. He is determined to find the reason for this increase in customer dissatisfaction and decides to carry out an audit. James is aware that there are

continued overleaf

many factors that could affect the time taken for prescriptions to be completed. One factor that he is particularly interested in is the level of staffing at different times of the working day. He plans to construct an audit to determine the number of staff available for the dispensing process at different times of the day and some indication of their skill level. The information he gains from this audit helps him to identify certain problem areas that relate to staff management and training. Some of these problem areas could be improved by more proactive management of staff, and he identifies this as an area for CPD.

Critical reflection on the information provided by an audit can act as a stimulus to help identify individual learning needs.

Reading and continuing education events

Active reading of journal articles and the participation in CE activities such as workshops can often encourage the wider exploration of an area of personal development. The consideration of questions such as those found in the 'Checkpoint' sections at the start of the chapters in this book can be a useful tool. The questions can act as a prompt to ask: 'Is this subject relevant to my practice and how can I apply this knowledge?'

Example 1.4

James attends a local Centre for Pharmacy Postgraduate Education (CPPE) evening on hypertension, and in the pre-course reading and during the presentation there is reference to the taking of accurate blood pressure readings. He already supplies digital blood pressure meters and would like to offer a blood pressure monitoring service. However, the practical use of blood pressure meters and obtaining an accurate reading is not covered in the workshop. It is some time since he was involved in taking blood pressure readings and he feels that his knowledge and level of skill in this area must be improved if he were to introduce a blood pressure monitoring service.

Being prompted by organisational priorities

In some cases the reflection may be imposed from above, through an employer or by the implementation of national priorities by a local primary care organisation (PCO).

Example 1.5

The pharmacy multiple that employs James decides that his pharmacy is to start offering a cholesterol testing service within the next 6 months. James starts to reflect on the knowledge and skills needed to be able to deliver this service. The company training department has produced a training manual designed to prepare all staff for the launch of this new service. James quickly skims through the training material and aims to focus on areas that he feels less confident in. For example he has recently read some articles on hypercholesterolaemia and feels confident to be able to discuss total cholesterol readings and associated risk factors. However, he is much less confident about the practical aspects of taking blood samples and interacting with the client in a more clinical setting. On reflection he decides that this is the area that he needs to develop and gain confidence in.

Being prompted by local and national policies

National priorities and specific local initiatives can sometimes prompt the individual pharmacist to think more clearly about their CPD needs.

Example 1.6

The NSF for Older People highlights the issue of falls in the elderly.[11] James's local PCO will be shortly introducing a project to reduce the incidence of falls in older people. This programme involves a domiciliary visit by the local pharmacist to assess the medication of patients identified by other healthcare professionals as at risk of falls. James would like to become involved in this project and starts to reflect on the knowledge and skills needed to carry out the medication assessment. As part of his reflection he starts to list the types of medication

continued overleaf

associated with falls in older patients, and draws out a flow diagram of some of the issues involved. He finds this exercise relatively straightforward and feels that he has the necessary clinical knowledge in this area. However, he does not feel as confident in conducting a patient interview and has not been involved in a domiciliary visit of this type before. James makes a telephone enquiry about the project to express his interest and voice his reservations. The local project lead assures him that a full induction process is available, which includes interview observation and work shadowing. He decides that involvement in this project would provide the opportunity to develop his patient interview skills.

Reflecting on RPSGB areas of competence

Another approach is to regularly take stock of our competence by matching our own self-assessed competence against published criteria.

Example 1.7

James logs on to the RPSGB Plan and Record website,[12] and browses through the key areas of competence (Appendix 7). He looks at the areas of competence specific to community pharmacy. This list acts as a prompt for reflecting on his own CPD. He decides by looking at the list that he would like to prioritise a key area of competence that would benefit his practice as a pharmacist. Recently he has had some queries from a local nursing home about waste disposal, which he has been unable to answer. Looking at the list of areas of competence he notices that 'Disposing of medication and participating in medicine disposal schemes' (competence C6g) comes under the broader heading of: 'Supplying medicines, dressings and appliances; and managing stock'.

James decides that his working knowledge of waste disposal legislation is not up to date and is inadequate. By looking at this list of areas of competence it has prompted him to reflect on his own CPD in this area. He decides he will return to this list of competences to reflect on his practice in other areas.

Having looked at different opportunities to reflect on practice we now need to set specific learning objectives. The SMART acronym is a useful tool when setting objectives.

- *S – specific*: the objective should state clearly what it is that you want to be able to do.
- *M – measurable*: will it be possible to determine if you have met your learning objective?
- *A – achievable*: will it be possible to achieve your objective when you take into account resources such as time, cost and support?
- *R – relevant*: is the learning objective relevant to your practice? The more specific your objective, the more useful it is likely to be. Avoid using woolly or broad statements.
- *T – timed*: your specific objective needs a specific deadline for your goal to become real.

Using the specific examples, James Brown could now set learning objectives to be achieved within a set time period:

- *Example 1.1*: to be aware of the current evidence base for glucosamine products and be able to summarise this for interested customers
- *Example 1.2*: to introduce a user-friendly hard copy filing system that will assist him in his response to customer queries
- *Example 1.3*: to introduce a new staff hours management system that takes into account skill mix and the needs of the business at different times of the day
- *Example 1.4*: to demonstrate the ability to take an accurate blood pressure reading and to confidently discuss all the different types of digital blood pressure meters
- *Example 1.5*: to be able to competently perform a test for total cholesterol within specified guidelines
- *Example 1.6*: to be able to confidently conduct a structured patient interview
- *Example 1.7*: to be able to brief the pharmacy team on the correct procedures for the collection and disposal of pharmacy waste.

We are now in a position to move to the next stage of the cycle, which is the planning of our CPD.

Planning

In the examples of the previous section, specific learning needs have been identified. The next stage is to prioritise these learning needs and make a decision on how these needs will be met. Many of the skills needed in planning CPD such as time management and prioritising needs will be covered in Chapter 2.

The first part of the planning stage is to decide on the urgency of the identified objectives. There may be an urgent and immediate need to meet an identified objective or the objective may relate to an ongoing

Table 1.1 CPD planning: assessment of different learning methods

Learning objective: to improve my management skills by the introduction of a new staff hours management system that takes into account skill mix and the needs of the business

Proposed activity	Advantage	Disadvantage
Experiment by introducing a new timetable of staff working hours and see how this works in practice	Quick to implement	Not obtaining any external input and there could possibly be serious consequences and human resource issues if the proposal does not work in practice
Speak to a colleague in another pharmacy who has a good system of tracking staff hours using IT, and ask them for advice	Gaining the insight and experience of a colleague that appears to be well organised and has introduced a system that works well in practice	Finding time for a meeting to discuss the system at length and decide if it would be appropriate for the situation
Select assessed modules of a management skills course that involves assertiveness training and how to successfully introduce change	Obtaining expert opinion on this specific dilemma and addressing the key issue, i.e. the introduction of change into the culture of a well-established pharmacy working pattern	May eventually have the knowledge to carry out the change successfully but the process of studying modules and being assessed will be onerous and take a long time to complete

development need that will only become apparent over a period of months or years. For example the provision of a cholesterol-testing service (Example 1.5) is to take place within the next 6 months and so there is not an immediate need to meet this learning objective. The objective relating to glucosamine (Example 1.1) is much more urgent as local GPs are now starting to prescribe or recommend this product.

The second stage of the planning process is to consider the importance of the learning objective in terms of how the learning will impact on yourself, your colleagues, your organisation and your service users.

In one of the previous examples, the development of management skills and the introduction of a new staff hours management system (Example 1.3) is important as this is already impacting on levels of service and ultimately patient care. When assessing the importance of a learning objective the pharmacist needs to stand back and ask the question: 'How often will I use the new skill or knowledge in my practice?' The management skills required in this example will have high importance as this skill is used every day in the management of staff. The other examples all involve skills or knowledge that are likely to be used less frequently. It is only by looking at the urgency and importance attached to a learning objective that each one can be prioritised and a date set to achieve the objective. It is always necessary to set a specific date when writing a SMART objective.

Having identified the urgency and importance of the task it is now necessary to identify appropriate activities to meet the learning needs. There are many different ways of meeting objectives. Ideally a wide variety of options are considered that take into account the individual preferred learning style and the resources available. In the initial stages it is useful to note the activities that are considered to be the most appropriate and then systematically look at the advantages and disadvantages of each method. This process may seem quite time consuming but ensures that the time and effort is invested in the most appropriate learning activities. An example of assessing different learning methods for meeting an objective is summarised in Table 1.1

By looking at the advantages and disadvantages we are in the position to make a professional judgement about the best course of action. Action is the next stage of the CPD cycle.

Action

This part of the CPD process is about implementing plans that have been selected during the planning stage.

Example 1.8 Extract from James Brown's CPD record

After speaking to my colleague about his system of managing staff working hours I can now use a piece of software to construct a working hours matrix that relates to skill level, volume of business and staff availability. My colleague has offered to look at the initial draft of my revised schedule of staffing before I implement it, which I hope to do in the next week.

The specific plans are carried out within the defined time limit and a summary is made of what has been achieved. Once the planned activity has taken place, it is time to move on to the evaluation stage.

Evaluation

At this stage of the CPD cycle, questions are being asked such as:

- has my learning objective been met?
- have I tested if what I have learnt can be applied to practice?
- am I now able to work differently?
- were there any problems with the reflection, planning or action parts of the CPD cycle? (For example was the learning need identified correctly and the objective specific enough?)

Example 1.9 Extract from James Brown's CPD record

My colleague thought my initial draft needed amending to take into account the need for more dispensary staff on a Saturday morning. I followed this suggestion and have introduced the new programme of working hours. Generally the new system has worked well and this has encouraged me to look more closely at staff working hours. However, I have found it difficult to introduce these changes as staff members seem very unwilling to change their hours and this has caused some ill feeling. Increased Saturday working has been particularly unpopular and I feel that I need further development of my management skills to be able to carry through this change successfully.

This is an example where the CPD cycle would be re-entered at reflection to pinpoint what particular management skills are needed to address this ongoing problem.

Unscheduled learning

Not all CPD falls into the neat cycle of reflection, planning, action and evaluation. In some cases the pharmacist may have a conversation with a colleague or attend a training event and learn something that could be applied specifically to their practice. The learning is unscheduled or opportunistic as it was not a planned piece of CPD.

This type of learning starts with action and moves on to the evaluation of what was learnt. In some cases this may be developed further by reflecting in more depth and moving on to the reflection stage of a new CPD cycle.

Example 1.10

James Brown reads an article in the *Pharmaceutical Journal* on the treatment of fungal nail infections and studies the additional advice that should be given to patients with a fungal nail infection to prevent recurrence. James notes the importance of this advice in achieving a successful long-term outcome for the patient. This prompts him to think about his knowledge and practice when giving additional advice for other fungal infections such as athlete's foot and vaginal candidiasis. James starts to develop a series of additional advice protocols for use within the pharmacy team when speaking to patients with fungal infections.

Plan and record

The pharmacist CPD record should comply with the good practice criteria published by the RPSGB. Good practice criteria and useful advice to support the pharmacist in recording their CPD are available on the RPSGB Plan and Record section of the CPD website.[12] Referring to these criteria can help to ensure that the CPD portfolio is balanced. It is important that a CPD record includes examples of learning that starts at action, and learning that starts at reflection.

The CPD portfolio can be documented either on paper and retained in a file, or recorded electronically by making a website entry. The format is the same in either case and copies of exemplar record sheets can be seen on the Plan and Record website. Electronic recording of CPD is the preferred option as there is easy access to additional information at the time of entering the online record. The web-based record is also more secure than a paper version which could be mislaid or destroyed.

Current guidance is that it should take approximately 30 minutes to record one CPD entry and approximately one entry should be made each month. The pharmacist may choose to engage in much more CPD than this, depending on their personal circumstances and development needs. The aim of CPD recording is to produce a portfolio of good-quality entries. The portfolio should reflect good practice criteria, using different learning activities, rather than a large collection of similar entries.

Once the initial hurdle of the first entry has been made and the user becomes familiar with the recording procedure, the process becomes more integrated into working practice. Ultimately the individual CPD programme is driven by and linked closely to individual personal development planning.

Personal development planning

CPD that is unplanned and spontaneous is unlikely to bring about the maximum return in terms of your investment of time and effort. A PDP is essentially a plan of action. The PDP provides the pharmacist with the opportunity to set personal targets and find the best way to achieve these targets. A well constructed PDP takes a more global view of where the pharmacist is heading and what they would like to achieve along the way. Different formats can be used for a PDP. The RPSGB has a pro forma that can be used and asks a series of questions to help establish CPD priorities. Alternatively, the pharmacist may prefer to use a different format or construct their own PDP. The following stages are required to produce a PDP.

A PDP is based on three questions:

- where am I now?
- where do I want to be?
- how can I get there?

Where am I now?

Asking this general question will lead to additional questions such as:

- what am I good at?
- what do I need to work on?
- what could help me overcome my weak areas?
- what could be a barrier to the change I need to make?

At this stage the lower edge of the development gap is being defined.

Where do I want to be?

This is a very personal question and there will be many variables to consider in formulating your answer. The questions listed below may help to answer the question. It will be necessary to ask many other questions to formulate an answer to this question. For example:

- what do I like doing?
- what is my motive for personal development?
- what is my ultimate personal/professional goal?
- how will I measure my success?

It may be easier to answer this question in stages by setting a series of goals to reach the final endpoint rather than one massive goal that seems unrealistic.

By answering this question the upper limit of the development gap is being defined.

How can I get there?

Having identified the development gap the next stage is to determine how your objective can be achieved. An effective PDP will consist of a number of manageable portions in order to achieve the overall aim. The plan for achieving a development goal will ideally consist of short-, medium- and long-term objectives. PDPs are not set in stone and need to be reviewed regularly. For example a PDP may include short-term goals to be reviewed in 3 months' time, medium-term goals to be reviewed in 6 months and a long-term goal to be reviewed after 2 years. Different timeframes need to be selected that will be suitable for both the individual and the organisation that the individual is associated with. When asking the question 'how can I get there?' it is important to be realistic about factors that will affect progress. Remember to factor social, domestic, monetary and organisational constraints into the objectives. Keep your objectives SMART.

Figure 1.3 provides a summary diagram of the basic structure of a PDP.

The PDP should not be set in stone but is a fluid and evolving document as individual circumstances and aspirations change.

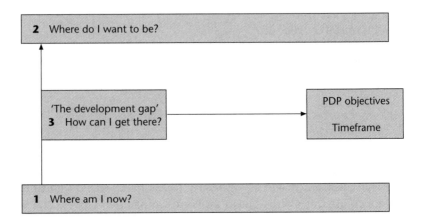

Figure 1.3   Constructing a personal development plan.

Example 1.11   Personal development plan

Anita Taylor qualified as a pharmacist 3 years ago. The first two years of practice she worked for a large multiple as a relief pharmacist. Anita then spent 6 months self-employed as a locum pharmacist before moving to her current position as the pharmacist-manager of a busy pharmacy that is part of a small multiple group.

Extracts from Anita Taylor's PDP planning notes
Where am I now?
Some recent workplace incidents that have added to my sense of job satisfaction:

- performed first MUR [medicines use review] on a patient and felt that it went well and felt comfortable in this role
- Recently tutored an enthusiastic summer vacation student and found that I really enjoyed discussing responding to symptoms and different over-the-counter (OTC) medicines that have recently been deregulated from POM [prescription only medicine] to P [pharmacy medicine]. I found it beneficial being able to discuss this in more detail and found that by having to explain this area it improved my own knowledge.

Learning needs that have arisen from these experiences
Although I found these experiences increased my sense of job satisfaction I wish my clinical knowledge was more up to date. The MUR patient asked some searching questions about their angina and I feel

→

that it would be useful to update my clinical knowledge in this area. The informal tutoring of a vacation student was useful as I have not been involved in this type of work before. I feel that my tutoring and coaching skills could be improved as I would like to act as a preregistration tutor next year.

Workplace issues that will impact on my PDP

- There is a large amount of pressure to increase the amount of business with residential homes and there is the strong possibility that my store will be a centralised point for this business.
- The company is aiming to introduce a new PMR [patient medication record] system next year. The system will facilitate the recording of much more information and will enhance my clinical role further.
- I have seen a peripatetic pharmacist training position advertised that will involve delivering off the job training sessions for all levels of pharmacy staff. I would be very interested in this type of work.

Local issues that will impact on my PDP
The local PCO is trying to engage pharmacists in a new domiciliary visiting scheme and medicines management service with the elderly.

Where do I want to be? Career plans for the next 3–5 years
I would like to achieve the following:

- a clinical diploma qualification with an emphasis on community pharmacy and offering enhanced services
- be able to offer a medicines management service to care homes and develop expertise in this area
- tutor a preregistration graduate
- develop my tutoring and clinical skills
- be in a strong position to apply for a future pharmacist training role when this is advertised.

How do I get there? Personal development plan outline
Objectives – Year 1
(Review every 3 months. A PDP should have specific review dates so that the pharmacist can work towards achieving each specific goal.)

- Research suitable clinical diploma courses that have a community pharmacy bias. Look at flexibility of modules and types of assessment and possibility of funding from employer. Select a course that fulfils criteria and start the course at the next available opportunity.

continued overleaf

- Arrange meeting with manager to discuss personal development and express interest in training and future development opportunities. Offer willingness to work as a preregistration tutor for the next year.
- Arrange meeting with primary care pharmacist to discuss opportunities locally and offer to become involved in domiciliary visiting scheme.
- Undertake the necessary training to become accredited to offer medication management service to care homes. Undergo CPD activities to ensure that I am competent in this area.

Provisional objectives could be written for year 2 at this stage, or the objectives could be written later in the first year in line with how the PDP is evolving.

Top tips for producing a PDP

- *Think positive*: the production of a PDP should be an exciting prospect as it is all about what could be possible and achievable.
- *Think about the future*: the challenge is to stay current in our own field of expertise. To achieve this requires forward planning.
- *Find a mentor*: this person needs to be non-judgemental and willing to offer help by providing feedback, suggestions and a support framework. For the pharmacist that works alone a mentor is particularly important as it is often difficult to assess in isolation how your PDP is progressing.
- *Make full use of all resources available*: resources include the internet, increasing quantities of literature and training materials and the expertise of colleagues. All of these resources can input into a PDP.
- *Take a broad pragmatic approach when developing a PDP*.

The pharmacist with a PDP has a powerful tool to develop professional and personal expertise in a systematic way. Producing a PDP is a vital step in your professional life – a blueprint for the future that may change the course of your life journey.

Implications for practice

Activity 1

Carry out a review of your CPD entries over the past 6 months using the RPSGB pro forma (Personal Review of CPD Record, RPSGB website, Appendix 5).

- Do you see any patterns emerging in the way that you write your CPD entries?
- Is it clear what you have both learnt and applied over the past 6 months?
- Will this exercise make your next CPD entries different in any way?

Activity 2

Using a blank sheet of paper write a first draft of your own PDP for the next year using the questions: 'Where am I now?' 'Where do I want to be?' 'How do I get there?'

Multiple choice questions

Directions for questions 1 and 2: each of the questions or incomplete statements in this section is followed by five suggested answers. Select the best answer in each case.

Q1   Which one of the following most closely matches the function of the Healthcare Commission?

A   Setting National Service Frameworks
B   Setting clinical standards
C   Monitoring standards in the NHS
D   Monitoring participation in CPD for healthcare professionals
E   Improving patient and public involvement in healthcare

Q2   Which of the following most clearly represents the CPD cycle?

A   Evaluation, action, reflection, planning
B   Planning, reflection, evaluation, action
C   Action, planning, evaluation, reflection
D   Reflection, planning, action, evaluation
E   Reflection, action, evaluation, planning

Directions for questions 3 to 6: for each numbered question select the one lettered option above it which is most closely related to it. Within each group of questions each lettered option may be used once, more than once, or not at all.

Questions 3 and 4 refer to different stages of the CPD cycle.

A   All stages of the CPD cycle
B   Evaluation
C   Action
D   Planning
E   Reflection

A pharmacist observes that there is a clinical article on the treatment of hypertension in the *Pharmaceutical Journal*. Select from A to E which one of the above fits the following statements.

Q3   After reading the article and the suggested additional reading the pharmacist asks the question: 'Am I now able to work differently?'
Q4   A pharmacist decides not to read the article as he already has the theoretical knowledge in this subject area but is looking for training to improve his practical skills in this area.

Questions 5 and 6 are about the following documentation:

A   Bristol Royal Infirmary Inquiry (Kennedy report)[1]
B   *The NHS Plan*[2]
C   *Pharmacy in the Future*[13]
D   RPSGB Code of Ethics[5]
E   RPSGB 'Plan and Record'[12]

Which of the following statements most closely matches the document?

Q5   A requirement for all practising pharmacists to adopt CPD.
Q6   A recommendation that all healthcare professionals should undergo appraisal, CPD and revalidation as part of their contract.

Directions for questions 7 and 8: each of the questions or incomplete statements in this section is followed by three responses. For each question ONE or MORE of the responses is (are) correct. Decide which of the responses is (are) correct. Then choose:

A   if **1, 2** and **3** are correct
B   if **1** and **2** only are correct
C   if **2** and **3** only are correct
D   if **1** only is correct
E   if **3** only is correct

Directions summarised:
A: 1, 2, 3   B: 1, 2 only   C: 2, 3 only   D: 1 only   E: 3 only

Q7   This question is about continuing education (CE)

1   CE is often specific for individual pharmacists and their development needs.
2   CE often has a passive approach to learning.
3   CE assessment is often knowledge based.

Q8   Which of the following are ways of reflecting on practice as a community pharmacist?

1   Critical incident analysis

2   Professional audit
3   Peer review

Directions for questions 9 and 10: The following questions consist of a statement in the left-hand column followed by a second statement in the right-hand column.
Decide whether the first statement is true or false.
Decide whether the second statement is true or false.
Then choose:

A   if both statements are true and the second statement is a correct explanation of the first statement
B   if both statements are true but the second statement is NOT a correct explanation of the first statement
C   if the first statement is true but the second statement is false
D   if the first statement is false but the second statement is true
E   if both statements are false

Directions summarised:

A:	True	True	second statement is **a correct explanation** of the first
B:	True	True	second statement is **NOT a correct explanation** of the first
C:	True	False	
D:	False	True	
E:	False	False	

Q9   As part of their CPD a newly registered pharmacist sets the following objective: 'To become accredited to offer a medicines use review service in the pharmacy using the CPPE online assessment within the next two months'.

■   *Statement 1*: The objective is not specific and needs to be rewritten.
■   *Statement 2*: The SMART acronym is a useful tool when setting objectives.

Q10

■   *Statement 1*: When planning CPD it is necessary to list as many options as possible to fulfil a specific learning need and look at the advantages and disadvantages of each option.
■   *Statement 2*: When planning CPD it is important that a wide variety of options are considered that take into account the individual learning style of the pharmacist and ensure that time is invested in the most appropriate learning.

Case studies

Level 1

John is a pharmacy undergraduate in year 2 of the MPharm degree course. He is fairly quiet and can sometimes appear aloof and reserved. He has enjoyed the pharmaceutical science modules but has found the pharmacy practice part of the course more challenging. John feels especially uncomfortable when working as part of a group or being asked to make a formal presentation to his colleagues. He has no previous experience of working in a pharmacy and tends to spend his holidays travelling and working part-time in an accounts office. He is very unsure about where to apply for his preregistration training but was quite interested in a presentation on hospital pharmacy recently held at the university. At a recent meeting with his tutor he was asked to write a brief statement for his personal development portfolio, including some personal objectives for the next year.

- Write four objectives for John to include in his portfolio that could be achievable over the next year.

Level 2

John is now a preregistation graduate working in a hospital pharmacy department. The preregistration year has been challenging and there have been times when he has found it difficult to work with some other members of staff, especially pharmacy technicians. The registration exam is now only 4 months away and he is working hard to ensure he has covered all the necessary parts of the exam syllabus. In his last appraisal meeting his tutor expressed the view that she had some concerns relating to his communication skills. He has decided that once registered he would like to work in community pharmacy. He does not wish to pursue a career in hospital pharmacy at this stage. He has recently seen a vacancy for a pharmacist-manager in his home town that would be ideal for his personal circumstances.

He has obtained the following information about the vacancy:

- town centre pharmacy, part of a small multiple and dispenses approximately 600 items per week. Pharmacy located on a busy road with inadequate space for parking
- main competition is a well-managed health centre pharmacy that is about 100 m away

- business has been managed by a series of locum pharmacists for over 9 months
- would consider newly qualified pharmacist and there is some induction training available
- staff team well established and reasonably motivated and includes a qualified pharmacy technician
- the owner is keen to develop the business further and to participate in the provision of new pharmacy services.

John decides to apply for the position. As part of the application process he is required to produce a short statement outlining his personal and professional development needs.

- Using SMART objectives outline a personal development plan for John *before* he starts work as a community pharmacist in his first pharmacy.

Level 3

John was offered the position and has been in post for 6 months. He has an informal meeting with his employer to discuss his work. His employer is pleased with how John has settled into the business and has noted the positive increase in prescription volume and turnover. He is keen for John to expand the business and to be able to offer a supply and advisory service to residential homes. John agrees to this in principle but needs to undertake some CPD in this area. Later that week John reflects on this area and starts to complete the RPSGB documentation for a new CPD cycle.

- Outline the *reflection* and *planning* sections of John's CPD entry.

References

1   *The Bristol Royal Infirmary Inquiry – Final Report* (2001). www.bristol-inquiry.org.uk/ (accessed 24 August 2007).
2   Department of Health. *The NHS Plan: a plan for investment a plan for reform.* London: Department of Health, 2000. www.dh.gov.uk/en/Publicationsandstatistics/Publications/PublicationsPolicyAndGuidance/DH_4002960 (accessed 24 August 2007).
3   Hunt P. *Pharmacy in the Future – Implementing the NHS Plan.* London: The Stationery Office, 2000.
4   Royal Pharmaceutical Society of Great Britain (RPSGB). *Pharmacy in a New Age.* London: RPSGB, 1995.
5   Royal Pharmaceutical Society of Great Britain. *Code of Ethics for*

Pharmacists and Pharmacy Technicians. London: Royal Pharmaceutical Society of Great Britain, 2007.

6   Institution of Civil Engineers. *Continuing Professional Development ICE 3006.* www.ice.org.uk/downloads/ICE3006_ContinuingProfessional Development.pdf (accessed 24 August 2007).

7   Department of Health. *Clinical Governance: quality in the new NHS* (HSC 1999/065) London: Department of Health, 1999.

8   Fraser S, Greenhalgh T. Coping with complexity: educating for capability *BMJ* 2001; **323**: 799–803.

9   Attewell J, Blenkinsopp A, Black P. Community pharmacists and continuing professional development – a qualitative study of perceptions and current involvement. *Pharm J* 2005; **274**: 519–524.

10   Mottram DR, Rowe P, Gangani N, Al-Khamis Y. Pharmacists' engagement in continuing education and attitudes towards CPD. *Pharm J* 2002; **269**: 618–622.

11   Department of Health. *National Service Framework for Older People.* London: Department of Health, 2001. www.dh.gov.uk/en/Publications andstatistics/Publications/PublicationsPolicyAndGuidance/DH_400306 6 (accessed 7 September 2007).

12   Royal Pharmaceutical Society of Great Britain. *CPD for Pharmacists and Pharmacy Technicians in Great Britain.* www.uptodate.org.uk/home/ PlanRecord.shtml (accessed 24 August 2007).

13   Department of Health. *Pharmacy in the Future: implementing the NHS Plan. A programme for pharmacy in the National Health Service.* London: Department of Health, 2000. www.dh.gov.uk/en/Publicationsand statistics/Publications/PublicationsPolicyAndGuidance/DH_4005917 (accessed 7 September 2007).

2

Management skills in the pharmacy

Failing organisations are usually over-managed and under-led.
                                                    (Warren G Bennis)

Checkpoint

Before reading on, think about the following questions to identify
your own knowledge gaps in this area:

- What are the principles of effective meetings management?
- How does a successful team differ from a group of workers?
- Give one example of a simple time-management tool.
- Describe one theory of motivation in the workplace. How could I
  apply this theory to the pharmacy team?

Many advertisements for pharmacist positions in community pharmacy
are for the job title of pharmacist-manager. Even within the more clinically
orientated positions, the community pharmacist will be expected to manage clearly defined projects that will call on their management skills. This
dual role of both pharmacist and manager can sometimes cause conflict as
the pharmacist may struggle to effectively balance the two roles. In many
cases, the pharmacist will focus on their professional role and neglect their
management responsibilities. This unbalanced approach can often lead to
reduced job satisfaction. Increasingly the specific management skills
required by the community pharmacist are necessary in order to participate
more fully in their professional role. This chapter focuses on the management skills required in the community pharmacy in order to be effective in
offering new services. The implementation of new services makes new
demands on our resources and the way that the pharmacy team operates.
Before new services can be launched it is necessary to look at how established management techniques can help to achieve our objectives.

In many cases the community pharmacist has unusual working conditions compared to other managers. This is often a consequence of the
high level of public accessibility and the pharmacist being actively
engaged in the supply process.

The Health Act 2006 addresses many of the difficulties relating to the requirements about supervision and responsibility in a community pharmacy. The Health Act replaces the more rigid requirement for 'personal control' with the provision of a 'responsible pharmacist'. The 'responsible pharmacist' will have professional accountability for all processes in the pharmacy. This would allow the pharmacist to be temporarily absent from the pharmacy to engage in such activities as meetings with general practitioners (GPs) or offering services to patients in their own home. This legislation also permits the appropriate delegation of the supervision of the sale and supply of medicines to trained registered pharmacy technicians, without the direct supervision of a pharmacist. This is designed to enable the pharmacist to use their skills more effectively and offer a wider range of services.

The specific practical details of these changes are not set out in the legislation but are to be formulated into regulations. At the time of writing, work was in progress on the new regulations to be made under the Act that relate to the 'responsible pharmacist' and 'supervision'.

It is anticipated that the regulations should clearly define those activities that can only be undertaken when the responsible pharmacist is present. The detail of any delegation should include clear lines of accountability and a robust system of being able to contact the responsible pharmacist when they are absent from the pharmacy. As patient safety is a major concern, there would need to be a clear justification for the pharmacist being absent from the pharmacy and specific guidance on how remote supervision would operate in practice. It is clear that the new regulations will affect the framework in which the community pharmacist operates and will allow a much greater degree of flexibility.

This chapter aims to guide the community pharmacist through practical management methods specifically applied to a pharmacy environment. As an effective manager, the pharmacist is in a strong position to influence the quality of the services that they offer.

The Management Standards Centre, in response to studies showing that poor management is hindering the UK economy, has developed a set of standards for managers.[1] These standards were developed after extensive consultation with employers and individual managers. These management standards are used widely by many organisations within the UK and cover the main areas of:

- managing self and personal skills
- providing direction
- facilitating change
- working with people
- using resources
- achieving results.

Each area is divided into clear sections that can be used to self-assess individual skills and identify areas for continuing professional development. An overview of some of the management issues in a community pharmacy is outlined in Figure 2.1.

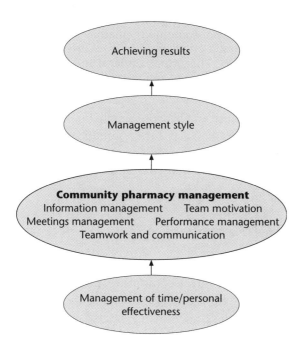

Figure 2.1 Overview of management issues in a community pharmacy.

Managing self and effective personal skills determine how successful the manager is in all other areas of management. The effective management of our time underpins all that we hope to achieve as a manager, particularly in the busy environment of a community pharmacy.

Time management

One of the frequent complaints of managers is that they have insufficient time to accomplish the tasks they have set out to achieve. Working in the community pharmacy setting can have specific frustrations compared to an office-based workplace. These differences need to be recognised at the outset, as many management theories can ignore the individual work setting and tend to apply the theory that one size fits all.

The community pharmacy manager has to overcome two specific problems in order to manage their time effectively:

- the pharmacist is available to patients at all times. The community pharmacist is probably the most accessible healthcare professional and can be accessed by a member of the public by telephone or by walking into a pharmacy and asking to speak to a pharmacist. Indeed this is one of the unique strengths of community pharmacy
- the pharmacist has traditionally been fully involved in the supervision of supplying medicines. This important legal and professional responsibility has taken priority and consumed a large proportion of working time.

These issues of availability and supervision are ones that are being actively debated and need to be addressed if the community pharmacist is to manage their time effectively. However, there are certain general principles that can be applied to ensure that your limited time is protected and used for maximum benefit.

General principles of time management

Commit to change

Time management starts with a commitment to change. It is about looking objectively about how time is used, making informed plans and carrying out our plans.

Time management is a skill that needs to be developed on an ongoing basis. It will involve making changes to our working practices and the relationships that we have with those we work with. The first step is to recognise that time management cannot be conquered in a day and will involve change.

Put first things first

One of the seven habits of highly effective people is to put first things first.[2] It is very easy to fill the day with routine tasks that are of secondary importance. Individuals and organisations need to focus on what matters most. Time management is about asking the question 'What is the most important issue?' The issue in question may be personal development, it may be providing a new service, it may be tackling an ongoing staff problem, or it may be dealing with a potentially difficult customer complaint. There are many areas that will call on our time, so our first task is to prioritise in terms of importance. This is not the same as asking if something is urgent or responding to the person who is shouting the loudest.

Use time-management tools

A useful time-management tool is to develop a matrix that determines if activities are urgent or important. An example of using this approach is outlined in Table 2.1.

Table 2.1   A time-management tool applied to a community pharmacy

Importance/ urgency	*Urgent*	*Not urgent*
Important	**A – do now** A dispensing error has been made and the patient is waiting to see you for an explanation. This would take full priority	**B – plan to do** Meet with practice manager of the local medical centre to discuss the new repeat dispensing service you are offering Plan space for important non-urgent tasks
Not important	**C – reject** A survey that will only take 'ten minutes of your time' and has to be completed in person now Reject impromptu activities such as these that demand your immediate attention but are not important. It is important to explain why you are rejecting this type of interruption	**D – resist** Read a journal article that does not relate to specific ongoing continuing professional development (CPD) Plan to avoid altogether any non-productive tasks that are neither important nor urgent

The effective time manager always asks the questions:

- is the task important?
- is the task urgent?

By assigning the task to a simple time-management matrix the manager is starting to plan their time and think about specific priorities.

Box A is for significant activities that have a real impact. It could include for example responding to the needs of a customer, a pre-arranged meeting, a serious staff issue or an imminent deadline for submitting a project proposal to the local primary care organisation. All of these could be classed as both important and urgent. It is possible that items that have been placed in Box B may now have A priority. For example the repeat dispensing service may have already been launched but you have not discussed this sufficiently with the practice staff and this will now potentially cause problems and so becomes an urgent and important task.

Box B is for planning and preparation. This is the area of the time-management matrix that is used to forward plan important meetings, develop new procedures or respond to staff or personal development needs. It is important to constantly review this area to check that the task is still important and that it has not moved to Box C.

Box C is for all the trivial and off-loaded requests from others. It covers a whole range of issues such as making duplicated effort or responding to unreasonable demands for information from staff or employers. These are activities that need to be rejected diplomatically and a careful explanation given as to why the task is being rejected. The explanation is important as this helps to generate a more open culture of how time is used and what is important in the management of the pharmacy. This is an area where the pharmacist aims to prevent re-occurrence of trivial demands. It may involve speaking to customers, suppliers, staff members and employers to look for a long-term solution to common urgent problem. For example if there is frequent questioning from staff on the medicine counter about a specific product, it may be useful to assign the issue to Box B and develop training material or a protocol that is going to ease the burden of future queries in this area.

Box D includes the activities that should be rejected completely. These include the endless possible interruptions to valuable time such as idle web browsing or allowing a customer to turn a professional consultation into an opportunity to chat. Pleasant as these activities are, they do not contribute to the proactive and effective completion of a daily work schedule. It is useful to ask for the reason behind Box D activities as sometimes they may be stress related and be seen as a release from the working day. The best antidote to such activities is to have a clear structure and schedule of tasks to the working day, which have been created in Box B. To do this will depend on the cultivation of good work habits.

Cultivate good work habits

Many of the tried and tested techniques for managing time are about cultivating good work habits. The following suggestions can be applied to the community pharmacy setting.

Keep a proper diary

The pharmacy diary needs to be a useful working tool and not become a task in its own right. This means that a clear and consistent system of diary keeping is in place that can be managed effectively. The use of a joint staff diary in a pharmacy is a useful time-planning tool. The type of diary will depend on individual preferences, and the merits of a traditional hard copy diary compared to an electronic diary need to be considered. One of the dangers of diary keeping is to use more than one document. This can be a real hindrance to time management and fragment the information that is needed to be able to make management decisions effectively. Ideally, the diary should be large enough to contain all the relevant information that will impact on the running of the pharmacy. Examples of this type of information include:

- all staff holidays
- times when local surgeries will be closed for staff development meetings
- potential busy times – for example by looking at the days before public holidays or local events.

By having this information accessible the manager is able to make both long-term plans (Box B-type activities) and short-term plans (Box A-type activities).

The diary can be clearly coded to ensure that if appointments are being made they are scheduled into the most appropriate time slot. For example if the pharmacy is offering a cholesterol-testing service by appointment it would seem practical to avoid booking any tests on the Friday before a bank holiday. The well-disciplined use of a diary by the entire pharmacy team ensures that there is a transparent working document that empowers the manager to make informed decisions.

Keep a 'to do' list

There is always the danger with 'to do' lists that the making of the list becomes an onerous task. The list should ideally be in electronic format that can be adjusted easily and quickly and tasks moved around as their priority changes. It is useful to keep a weekly overview of tasks that need to be completed and a daily 'to do' list with more detailed information. A useful format for a 'to do' list is provided in Table 2.2.

The daily 'to do' list is drawn from the weekly list and can only be written by taking into account the diary entries for that day. It is important that the list is fluid enough to take into account the needs of the business. The weekly list needs to be seen to be diminishing as the week progresses.

Table 2.2 Example format for a weekly/daily 'to do' list

To do – Week commencing ....

- Prepare for 39 week appraisal of prereg
- Complete pre-course reading for CPPE evening
- Finish off writing home visit reports – 8 to write
- Discuss new standard operating procedure for prescription reception with dispensing team
- Prepare for the contract visit from the PCT at the end of the month
- Ensure locum cover in place for trial extended opening hours next month
- Prepare presentation for local GPs to explain MUR service

Day	Diary entry	'To do'
Monday	Technician off on ACT training day, prereg on study leave (p.m.)	Prepare for 39 week appraisal of prereg Brainstorm ideas for presentation to GPs
Tuesday	Locum – all day a.m. – visit of area manager	a.m.: finalise preparation for area manager visit p.m.: write 4 home visit reports
Wednesday	Local surgeries closed half-day training day	p.m.: write 4 home visit reports Complete pre-course reading for CPPE evening
Thursday	a.m.: meeting with prereg to discuss calculations	p.m.: prepare meeting with staff to discuss new SOP for prescription reception – arrange suitable time for meeting (to take place before end of month) Start to prepare for the contract visit from the PCT at the end of the month – discuss audit form with senior technician – highlight areas that need to be acted on and agree action plan
Friday	Trainee disp (X) – annual leave	To do: discuss extended opening hours trial with staff and payments involved – set up voluntary rota system. Book pharmacist locum cover

ACT, accredited checking technician; CPPE, Centre for Pharmacy Postgraduate Education; PCT, primary care trust; SOP, standard operating procedure.

Do the most unpleasant job first

It is always tempting to tackle an easy task first. The theory behind this is that it will be achieved quickly and encourage the manager to go on and achieve more difficult tasks. First, if the task is very small and simple should a pharmacist-manager be doing it at all? Second, it is often the larger and more difficult task that is labelled as important that has clear business benefits.

As a pharmacist-manager you may be faced with a choice of two phone calls:

- phone a potentially difficult customer to discuss the options regarding the supply of a generic product that you are having difficulty sourcing
- phone a friendly regular customer to let them know some further information they requested about their new treatment.

The more difficult phone call is the starting point for the day. The difficult conversation cannot be postponed or the issue may escalate into a customer complaint and generate more work and involvement. Always start with more difficult tasks and use easier tasks as 'fillers' that can be done quickly at any time.

Eliminate distractions

A community pharmacy is a distracting place to work. There is a constant flow of people and conversation, ringing telephones and ad hoc queries. All of these distractions can deplete the positive energy required for tackling the major items on the 'to do' list. It is a useful exercise to devise ways of avoiding distraction. For example, consider the questions:

- what is a reasonable length of time for a telephone conversation?
- do some customers or members of staff make unreasonable demands on your time?
- is there any way that noise levels could be reduced?
- is it possible to make the pharmacy a less distracting place to work?

Remove clutter

Some pharmacy work areas are unnecessarily cluttered with a variety of papers, messages and 'post it' notes. In a dispensary working area this can be particularly hazardous where a clear flow of work is needed to provide an efficient service. Dispensary workflow is discussed further in Chapter 7. One effective work habit that will help to maximise time is to handle paper only once. Every day the post will include a variety of material ranging from circular junk mail to important communication giving details of product recalls. Ensure that a suitable filing system is in place so that the paper is not allowed to accumulate. Post opening should be done at a time when any item requiring action can be dealt with immediately. If any item of post requires a more detailed response the item should be annotated with a quick note and the task assigned to the weekly 'to do' list. The document should then be placed in a pending tray so that it can be located easily when the task is due. An accessible filing system should be used for all product information, letters and invoices, and items filed immediately where possible.

If there is an option to receive information electronically, always select this option to reduce the amount of paper that needs to be processed.

Analyse your time and work processes

Periodically it is worth while assessing the way that time is used for different tasks and the systems that operate in the pharmacy. This does not need to be an elaborate time and motion study but simply an indication of how the days are spent and how this correlates to your workload and staffing levels. Looking at systems and procedures with a critical eye is time well spent as it provides vital information on the efficiency of the pharmacy. This may involve looking at a practical area such as the most appropriate location for a dispensary stock item or a complex procedure for supplying a medicine under patient group directions.

Share your work

Where possible, work should be shared, especially if the task is large or tedious. For example making an inventory of controlled drugs for a stock audit is both quicker and easier if other members of the team are involved.

Seize the moment

Take every opportunity to use moments that are not actively engaged in work. (See Examples 2.1 below.)

Seek advice

If a pharmacist is planning a specific project there are often opportunities to seek advice from colleagues who have worked successfully on similar projects. Always ask for advice and cultivate sharing of ideas. Useful questions include:

Examples 2.1

- A pharmacist makes a telephone enquiry to a medical information department and is put on hold for several minutes. Many of the small tasks that have been allocated to the pending tray can be tackled in these short time slots.
- A staff member starts to talk informally to the pharmacist about an operational procedure that concerns them and this is part of a much wider issue that needs to be discussed as a team. The pharmacist uses the time to take proper notes of their concerns and files the record so that the time taken for the conversation is used to its full advantage.

- are there any short cuts that could be taken?
- are you on the right lines?
- have any important issues been overlooked?

By committing to change the way you work, putting first things first, using time-management tools and cultivating good work habits you are well on your way to conquering a skill that is in great demand – the effective use of time.

Motivating your team

A community pharmacist cannot achieve their work objectives in isolation. The pharmacist-manager depends on a co-operative, willing and able team in order to be able to meet deadlines and deal with difficult situations. In reality the manager may have to face employees who are tired, disgruntled and generally at odds with their working life. This is a difficult problem to overcome, particularly for the new manager who is enthusiastic about their role and finds it hard to accept the negativity of their pharmacy team. This section is about how to exert positive influence and motivate the pharmacy team.

A useful starting point is to consider your own behaviour and the impact it may have on your colleagues. Ask a few simple self-assessment questions:

- do I habitually moan about the work situation and the volume of work?
- do I complain about company procedures?
- do I act as a positive role model in offering a professional and positive experience for the customer?
- do I take time to explain what I am trying to achieve in my approach to work and in the ongoing development of the pharmacy?

- do I ensure that my team are frequently acknowledged for their contribution, and make reference to their successes?

It is by looking closely at our own behaviour that we start to realise the possible impact that we can have on the wider pharmacy team. The manager has to be motivated in order to be able to motivate a team. The first step to being a motivational manager is to be a positive role model.

The next step is to look at motivation as a long-term project rather than a quick easy fix. The pharmacy manager will need to develop an approach that is sustainable and maintains enthusiasm and commitment from their team. There are many different motivational theories that can be applied to the workplace. For this section we will confine the discussion to the 'Motivation–Hygiene' theory identified by Herzberg.[3] This theory is still widely accepted as an important piece of workplace psychology and can be applied to the pharmacy environment. Herzberg identified several factors such as salary levels, general working conditions and company policies which he called 'hygiene factors'. These factors can be demotivating if they are poor but do not tend to be motivating if they are good. For example if your pharmacy team works in a pharmacy that is in desperate need of a refit and staff are paid at the lower end of the salary scale and have to tolerate archaic company policies and procedures they will naturally feel demotivated. However, if all of these areas are addressed: the pharmacy is refitted to a high standard, their salary is improved to above the nearest competitor and the policies and procedures are streamlined, the pharmacy team will be more motivated. The theory suggests that once these factors have reached a certain standard, then further improvement will not motivate the workforce. The hygiene analogy is that once a workplace washroom is clean, no one cares if it is scrubbed up to an even higher standard of cleanliness.

The second part of Herzberg's theory involves looking at what people actually do in the workplace. The main motivators appear to be: a sense of achievement, recognition for work done, growth and advancement in their role and an interest in the job. In summary, additional monetary reward is pleasant but not as motivational as being valued and trusted.

To motivate a team, the manager needs to apply both hygiene and motivational factors simultaneously. The aim is to treat the team in the best way possible within the constraints of the organisation. This involves ensuring that the level of remuneration is competitive, the workplace environment is pleasant, the level of supervision and interpersonal relationships are satisfactory and there are seen to be sensible policies and procedures in place. Failure in these areas will lead to dissatisfaction. The challenge is to ensure that hygiene factors are in place and people are employed in such a way that they are able to achieve results, are recognised for what they do and are able to take responsibility for their work.

The pharmacist-manager who is keen to introduce the development of new services is in a strong position to be able to offer these motivational factors to the team.

For example, the introduction of an accredited checking technician (ACT) into the team provides the motivational opportunity for a suitable member of staff to be recognised, developed, valued and trusted.

When thinking about how to motivate a pharmacy team to achieve more, it is useful to ask the question: why do certain members of staff remain loyal and enthusiastic about their work? Many loyal members of pharmacy staff who remain in their work for many years feel stimulated by the healthcare environment in which they operate and their opportunity to contribute to the local community. Once the hygiene factors are in place, the manager's aim is to work on the motivational factors that are unique to the pharmacy environment.

Summary of pharmacy motivators

- *Achievement*: a motivational pharmacy manager takes the trouble to ensure that members of the team can achieve something tangible during their work. This will often lead to developing new skills and enhanced job satisfaction. For example, during a working week a new part of the patient medication record (PMR) programme is mastered or a team member is signed off as competent for a new standard operating procedure.
- *Recognition for achievement*: ensure that the efforts and achievements of the team are recognised; for example, the professional way a difficult customer is handled is acknowledged or success in a dispensing exam is celebrated.
- *Interest in the task*: this will mean taking the time on a regular basis to ensure that the type of work being done by team members is varied and, where possible, the task is put into context of the overall work. For example the member of staff recording the initial patient screening information for the supply of medication by patient group directions will have a much more positive approach to their work if they can see the importance of the questions they are asking. If they are unable to see the significance of the questions they will treat the task as a repetitive administrative exercise.
- *Give responsibility for the enlarged task*: by allocating responsibility for a discrete area of work, the tasks that make up that area can be seen as more palatable. For example, capping empty bottles to ensure that no dust collects in them is not the most exciting of tasks when faced with it in isolation every week. However, if this task is part of a much wider task of taking responsibility for all the packaging materials in the pharmacy including how and when they are ordered, stored and used, the motivation towards this task can change.

- *Growth and advancement to higher level tasks*: the manager will need an ongoing awareness of different levels of achievement of the pharmacy workforce, potential for increasing responsibility and succession planning. Individual team members will need encouragement so that they are working towards an appropriate level of achievement and are encouraged to engage in higher-level activities.

Management of meetings

Mismanaged meetings can be a time-wasting activity and costly in terms of resources and decreased staff morale. Conversely, a well-managed meeting that has been well thought out can be both productive and motivational. The holding of any significant meeting in a pharmacy can be difficult to achieve in normal working hours. This means that many meetings with the pharmacy team are informal and interrupted by the ongoing business of the pharmacy. Clearly this type of meeting is not ideal to discuss important business. If the meeting is held after a full working day it becomes especially important that the meeting is well planned to justify the time and cost involved for those attending. The pharmacist-manager will also need to attend meetings with other healthcare professionals, and in some cases will need to call their own meeting, for example when planning a new service. This section is designed to help the pharmacist manage meetings more effectively. The characteristics of a good meeting can be summarised under the headings listed below:[4]

- good preparation
- agreed procedures
- someone to lead, chair or support the meeting
- a focused discussion
- a clear purpose or agenda
- discussion of relevant matters
- effort to reach conclusions by consensus
- a forum for everyone to contribute
- each person is actively invited to contribute
- high-quality listening by everyone
- time managed
- rapid publication of results and further action.

The success of any meeting will depend on:

- careful input and preparation before the meeting
- appropriate actions and demeanour during and after a meeting
- continued evaluation after the meeting is over.

The stages involved in effective meetings management are summarised in Figure 2.2.

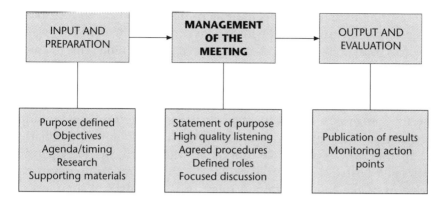

Figure 2.2 Stages involved in effective meetings management.

Before any meeting always ask the question: is this meeting necessary? If the main purpose of the meeting is to provide information then it may be that a meeting is not needed. If, however, the information being discussed is of a sensitive or controversial nature then a meeting may provide the opportunity for questions, comments and clarification. It would be unwise to circulate such information in a written memo or by email. Having established that a meeting is necessary, the next task is to undertake the important pre-meeting planning. The following summary is a useful checklist before the meeting:[5]

- clarify the purpose of the meeting and define objectives. These should be incorporated into the meeting documentation
- book the room, any audiovisual equipment and refreshments well in advance of the date of the meeting. Think about the most appropriate venue, as this should be neutral ground
- decide who should attend the meeting, based on who is most likely to contribute. It is important that the meeting is balanced and does not contain a majority of either over-dominating vociferous people or a significant group of introverted non-participants
- try to keep attendance at the meeting to a minimum
- organise and distribute a clear agenda and any supporting materials well in advance of the meeting
- schedule the meeting with clear start and end times and determine how long should be taken on each item of the agenda
- identify a chairperson; this does not necessarily have to be yourself.

Before the meeting the chairperson will need to consider the content of the meeting and the specific agenda items. By systematically working through the agenda items in advance, the chairperson is well prepared for the issues that may arise during the course of the meeting.

During the meeting it is the role of the chairperson to control the discussion and ensure that the meeting is conducted in an orderly way. It involves using well-developed observational and listening skills to ensure that all participants are involved. It is important to gain opinions from all present rather than let the loudest personality monopolise the meeting. The chairperson will also try and summarise and clarify the issues as the meeting progresses. This is for the benefit of the person taking minutes and also helpful to ensure that all participants are following the matters being discussed. In cases of confrontation where there are clear opposing views and heated discussion, it is useful if the chairperson reminds participants of pre-arranged ground rules for the conduct of the meeting. Sometimes it may be necessary to call for a break in the proceedings to diffuse a difficult situation. Minute writing involves recording the salient points regarding the discussion, and focuses on action to be taken by whom and when.

After the meeting ensure that the minutes are circulated within two weeks and monitor and evaluate the progress of the action points. This is a vital process for effective meetings management and ensures that the time spent on the meeting has been worth while.

Performance management

For many managers the term performance management can bring unsatisfactory images to mind such as conducting difficult appraisals and setting unrealistic targets. Performance management is a much broader activity that is all about getting the right things done successfully. The pharmacy manager is clearly a performance manager working towards achieving high standards of patient care through the performance of others. Management experts have tried to characterise performance management as either of two approaches:[6]

- *a process-based approach* which is based on a systematic analysis of the work done and the processes involved, in order to achieve the ideal predetermined result. Examples of this type of approach include operational research, job evaluation and management by setting objectives
- *a people approach* that works towards having the right people with the right skills in the right jobs and their effective management and motivation. Examples of this type of approach include training needs analysis, succession planning and performance-related pay.

In a community pharmacy the manager will be concerned with achieving the right skill mix and this is discussed further in Chapter 3. The manager will also be concerned with looking critically at systems of work and aiming to improve performance through detailed project planning.

Self-check questions for the pharmacist-manager

- Do I effectively communicate the vision of the pharmacy and the organisation so that the pharmacy team is aware of the current driving force behind what is trying to be achieved?
- Have I established key results, objectives and measures for the pharmacy business unit? These key results will not only be business based such as prescription volume but also relate to the provision and expansion of new services.
- Are there clearly identifiable business process objectives and key indicators of performance for those processes? For example a clearly defined procedure to identify patients suitable for a medicines use review (MUR) will translate into a key performance indicator of numbers of MURs completed each month.
- Have I identified key areas of the pharmacy business that I will need to monitor and evaluate?
- Is the performance of the pharmacy benchmarked against examples of good practice? Am I fully aware of quality indicators for a particular service?
- Do I keep myself informed of the performance of my competitors and, where there is a substantial shortfall in my activity, aim for concentrated improvement in performance?

Ultimately the performance of any pharmacy manager and the pharmacy team is measured by customers and service users. This is reflected in the use of customer satisfaction surveys within the pharmacy contractual framework.

Teamwork and communication

The traditional community pharmacist has tended to be seen as a lone worker with a strong directive management style. This independent image is at odds with the effective use of support staff and the building of a cohesive team. Making effective use of pharmacy support staff through appropriate levels of skill mix is considered instrumental to developing the pharmacist's role in delivering the government's medicines management agenda.[7] There has been much attention on skill mix issues for pharmacists and their support staff who work in the community and primary care sectors.[8] These issues will be explored further in Chapter 3 on training and development of the pharmacy team. It is important to note that even if the appropriate skill mix is in place and the number of hours of staffing is adequate, a pharmacy may under-perform through lack of a teamwork culture. A clear distinction can be made between a group and a team. Groups can be defined as two or more people who meet regularly over a period of time, perceive themselves as a distinct entity distinguishable from others, share common values and strive for common objectives.[9] The group of people working in a community pharmacy could easily fit into this definition. A team is also a group, but it takes on a much more sophisticated form. Teams are groups with complementary skills who are committed to a common purpose, clear performance goals, and approach to their work for which they hold themselves mutually accountable.[10] This collective way of working is more than putting together pieces of work in a co-ordinated manner; it is about team members being accountable for performance both as an individual member and as a team. This high ideal is much more difficult to achieve but has greater long-term rewards. In a community pharmacy culture that is rapidly changing, the isolated community pharmacist working with a group of support staff is no longer sustainable. The main characteristics of an effective team are outlined in Figure 2.3.

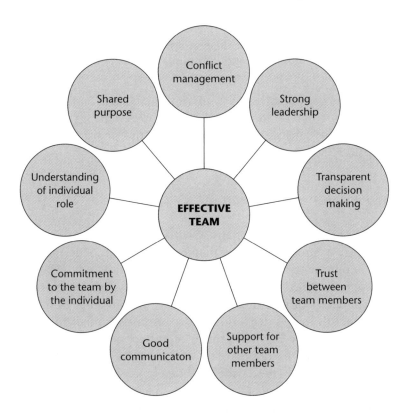

Figure 2.3   Characteristics of an effective team.

A successful pharmacy team needs a clear and well-communicated sense of purpose beyond surviving the everyday routine of inevitable tasks. The shared development of a mission statement gives focus to the priorities and activities of the team. The pharmacy team will need to identify their key areas of priority. For example a pharmacy may set up the following broad goals:

- to improve staff morale and systems of working
- to work more closely with other local healthcare professionals
- to build up strong relationships with customers.

Once the wider aims have been identified and agreed on, the next stage is to determine how team members will work towards the agreed ideal. This can be done by translating the goals into SMART (specific, measurable, achievable, relevant and timed) objectives and periodically measuring the success of the team. For example one specific team objective may be to ensure that all members of the dispensary team can readily identify all the GPs, practice nurses and receptionists at all the local medical centres. How this could be achieved and measured could be agreed by the team.

The Belbin team model is used by many organisations to analyse the way that their team works. Belbin defined a team role as being about how people behave in a team, how they contribute to a team and how they interrelate with other team members. He concluded that for a team to be balanced it should demonstrate nine different roles that are linked to personality types. An outline of Belbin's work and role descriptions can be found on the Belbin team roles website.[11] An individual leaning towards a particular role within a team can be determined by completing a Belbin questionnaire. This information can then be used to reflect on how the individual uses their role to contribute towards their team's effectiveness. One pitfall of using this type of approach is that the team member may become overly concerned with their Belbin role within the team. The team member may become unwilling to develop new ways of contributing to the team that they perceive to be outside their own area of strength. The Belbin system can be useful if a manager is setting up a new team as it provides the potential to include different types of team members. In practice many teams are already well established and will need to operate within the confines of the team members that they have. However, it can be useful for the established team to look at the way that it works together and the strengths of individual team members. The pharmacist is often expected to perform the role of team leader which equates to Belbin's co-ordinator role, even though this may be outside their own personality comfort zone.

Ideally a strong leader will:

- enable team members to become involved and committed to an agreed goal
- be an honest and open communicator
- celebrate success and achievement.

The issue of communication or lack of it is one that often causes problems in a team. In a community pharmacy where the team often works in close proximity, communication within the team should be a particular strength. Of all the many methods of communication including notice boards, memos, bulletins and email it is face-to-face contact and regular open dialogue that is the most effective. Regular praise and genuine encouragement are essential if a team is to flourish. Inevitably there will be times of conflict in any team and it is important to be able to deal with conflict issues speedily and effectively. Team problems should not be ignored, especially if other team members perceive that a team member is not contributing to an agreed team goal. For example, one method is to introduce a 'pharmacy problem log' which provides the transparent opportunity to report identified problems and look at how these can be resolved by requesting suggested solutions from the team. The log can be used to record all problem areas and assess work patterns that are emerging within the team.

It is well-recognised that successful teams enjoy their work and interact at a social level. It can be useful to arrange regular social events to ensure that the whole team has the opportunity to meet outside the working environment. Arranging a regular social event can have a positive impact on how the team interacts and communicates. It can be useful if the responsibility for organising the event is taken on by different members of the team.

One of the challenges for a manager is to build up an effective working team. Working as part of a successful team that communicates effectively can make the working environment a much more enjoyable place. This is a goal worth aspiring to for any pharmacist-manager.

Information management

In common with any manager, the community pharmacist will need to be able to manage information in order to make informed decisions. Information can be categorised according to its market value. The three main types of information can be classified as listed below:[12]

- *information for sale*: for example written material or software that is available at a market price. This often has a limited shelf life and its value declines with time, for example an externally produced and marketed information pack on how to set up a blood pressure monitoring service in your pharmacy

- *information that is freely available*: for example access to websites, pricelists, pharmaceutical advertisements and promotional material. In many cases, access to this type of material brings specific benefit to the owner of the information
- *information for internal use by an organisation* which is not intended to be sold and is of high value to the user. This includes business information, sales figures, prescription items, minutes of meetings and projected income from new services.

The pharmacist will use all the above types of information. However, it is the internal information that is of most value to the pharmacist-manager. As there is no external market for internal information, it is difficult to estimate the value of this type of information. The value of internal information is totally dependent on a number of factors such as:

- relevance
- completeness
- accuracy
- clarity
- timing.

Example 2.2

Moira Brown has managed a busy suburban pharmacy for over two years and is keen to develop new services. The following scenarios highlight the importance of information management in the pharmacy.

Scenario 1
Moira's projected sales figures for a new food allergy-testing service are very promising but are based on the figures from a pharmacy in a completely different demographic area to her own practice. She would need to question how relevant the figures are and if they could be applied to her own business.

Scenario 2
Moira wants to determine the best time to book MUR appointments so that she can have the appropriate staff resources in place to carry out this advanced service. She delegates a member of the dispensary team to collate information about staffing levels and prescription volumes. When the information is produced she realises that it does not present

continued overleaf

a complete picture as she has no information on all local surgery opening times and how many GPs are in surgery at any one time.

Scenario 3

Moira is pleased to notice a steady significant increase in prescription numbers over the past few weeks and starts to think how this will affect her staffing levels. On investigation she notices that there are some errors on the daily prescription record sheet entered by a new member of staff and realises that she is working with inaccurate information.

Scenario 4

The PMR system that Moira is using is adequate but does not always provide information in a clear and accessible form. To offer a more professional service and signpost patients to appropriate services she needs to be able to access collated information quickly and easily. Moira can foresee that she will need a more up-to-date system that will offer clear information and a means of engaging more fully in the new contract.

Scenario 5

Moira wishes to put in a proposal to offer a full pharmaceutical service to a 53-bed care home as she is aware that the home is about to change ownership. Moira is aware of some of the priorities of the new care home organisation and submits a detailed proposal to incorporate some of these priorities. Due to time pressures her proposal is not submitted until 3 months after the change of ownership, by which time the new owner has decided to take up the services of another pharmacy.

Using internal information and managing this information effectively is the lifeblood of any business. In common with many managers, the pharmacist can suffer from information overload.

Top tips for pharmacy information management

- Access your email inbox only at specific times of the day so that this does not interrupt your flow of work.
- Have a user-friendly hard copy filing system that will incorporate sections of information that can be easily accessed. Ideally, items should be filed immediately or placed in a designated filing tray. Examples of useful sections could include:
  - product information A–Z
  - patient information leaflets A–Z
  - primary care organisation (PCO) information

→

- health-promotion and signposting information
- prescribing information
- business information
- personnel files
- business development
- training and development.

■ Decide how information technology will be used to develop the pharmacy, and make a plan of how this will be achieved. Break down each requirement into manageable stages, for example: 'To become competent in the use of an electronic system of recording and referring MUR information'.

■ Look at ways of making appropriate business information clear, relevant and available to all of the pharmacy team. Consider regular short meetings to communicate information, and back this up with electronic and hard copies.

The successful pharmacist-manager will need to gain mastery over how they manage and use information. Knowledge and competence in the management of information will increasingly become an important characteristic of a successful community pharmacy manager.

Management style

The community pharmacist manager is usually responsible for a small team of people involved in the delivery of a safe and effective pharmaceutical service. Increasingly this will involve the delivery of patient-orientated pharmaceutical services. It is useful to reflect on your own individual management style and how this is influenced by your personality, and your working environment. Some management theories categorise managers into four basic types: directing, supporting, coaching and delegating.[13]

The directive management style can inspire confidence in your team and means that often you give clear and precise instructions. The disadvantage is that it can be seen as narrow and patronising and does not allow enough input from the team.

The supportive style of manager is good at giving feedback and an excellent listener. The disadvantage is that they can be seen to be swayed by too many opinions, and lacking in direction. The coaching manager uses a combination of directing and supporting and depends on building solid relationships within the team. Coaching will be discussed in more detail in Chapter 3. This vital skill can be applied to both the training and management of your staff. The delegating style of management will only work if there is clear communication about the delegated task. Many managers find it hard to let go of certain tasks and will only supervise rather than delegate. Other managers will be ineffective in their delegation of tasks as they will fail to follow up the initial delegation and be unclear about the outcome and the accountability for the task.

As a pharmacist you will need to employ all these different styles at different times and with different members of your team. The directive style may be more suitable to the medicine counter assistant that has just started and needs clear pointers about what they should be doing. A coaching style is appropriate to a trainee dispenser for example, who may have some well-developed skills but is unable to progress and lacks personal motivation. A combination of coaching and supervision can help to develop and manage this member of your team. A supporting style may be more appropriate when applied to a more mature member of the team that is very able but lacks confidence. By offering support and encouragement to take more responsibility the aim is to move this person on to a more independent state. The delegating style is most appropriate for example to an experienced and confident pharmacy technician. Provided the task, outcome and monitoring process are agreed in advance there is no reason why this member of staff cannot be delegated major objectives within the pharmacy, such as setting up a weight-management clinic or introducing a new system of repeat prescription collection.

Well-developed management skills are essential for the community pharmacist to engage fully in the new opportunities available in community pharmacy. An ongoing process for any manager is to reflect on some of the core management skills needed to make things happen within a pharmacy and link this with their ongoing continuing professional development (CPD).

Implications for practice

After reading this chapter are there any management skills that could be developed as part of your CPD?

Activity 1

Spend some time reflecting on how well the pharmacy team operates in your pharmacy. Which of the characteristics of an effective team:

- are evident?
- need more input and development?

Activity 2

Reflect on *two* different examples from your own practice where you have used different management styles. Was the management style used appropriate to the situation?

Directions for questions 1 and 2: each of the questions or incomplete statements in this section is followed by five suggested answers. Select the best answer in each case.

Q1 Time-management theory suggests all of the following *except*:

A   Using time-management tools such as a matrix that determine if a task is urgent or important
B   Always start with easier tasks that can be done quickly and removed from your 'to do' list
C   Eliminate distractions where possible
D   Spend time analysing your working day and work processes
E   Seek advice from others on their systems of work

Q2 According to Herzberg's theory the main motivators in a workplace are all of the following *except*:

A   Work that brings a sense of achievement
B   Recognition for work that is done
C   High level of remuneration
D   Career advancement
E   Genuine interest in the job

Directions for questions 3 to 5: for each numbered question select the one lettered option above it which is most closely related to it. Within each group of questions each lettered option may be used once, more than once, or not at all.

A   Co-ordinator
B   Shaper
C   Resource investigator
D   Plant
E   Team player

Select from A to E which one of the above fits the following statements.

According to the Belbin team profile:

Q3   A pharmacy technician who is very reflective and has excellent ideas but is unable to progress their ideas into a workable project.

Q4   A medicine counter assistant who is very outgoing and has a lot of contacts. They tend to quickly lose interest in a project once the initial enthusiasm has passed.

Q5   A challenging dispensing assistant who thrives under pressure and enjoys a challenge, particularly when there seem to be insurmountable obstacles. However, they can sometimes provoke other members of the team and may cause offence.

Directions for questions 6 to 8: each of the questions or incomplete statements in this section is followed by three responses. For each question ONE or MORE of the responses is (are) correct. Decide which of the responses is (are) correct. Then choose:

A   if **1**, **2** and **3** are correct
B   if **1** and **2** only are correct
C   if **2** and **3** only are correct
D   if **1** only is correct
E   if **3** only is correct

Directions summarised:
A: 1, 2, 3   B: 1, 2 only   C: 2, 3 only   D: 1 only   E: 3 only

Q6   The following statements are about information management:

1   There are three broad areas of information: information for sale, information that is freely available and internal information used by an organisation.

2   As a manager the most useful type of information is internal information.

3   Saleable information often has a limited shelf-life, and its value declines with time.

Q7   The following statements are about management styles:

1   A directive management style is often seen as positive and allows input from the pharmacy team.

2   A delegating management style is appropriate to a newly appointed medicine counter assistant.

3   A coaching management style uses a combination of directing and supporting management styles.

Q8   The following statements are about general management skills and their impact:

1   Managing self and the quality of a manager's interpersonal skills often determine how successful the manager is in all other areas of management.

2   The Management Standards Centre, after extensive consultation with
      employers and individual managers, developed a set of standards for
      managers that included such areas as: providing direction, using
      resources and achieving results.
3   The management skills of a pharmacist-manager will have a high
      impact on the quality of the services that they offer.

Directions for questions 9 and 10: The following questions consist of a
statement in the left-hand column followed by a second statement in the
right-hand column.
Decide whether the first statement is true or false.
Decide whether the second statement is true or false.
Then choose:

A   if both statements are true and the second statement is a correct
      explanation of the first statement
B   if both statements are true but the second statement is NOT a correct
      explanation of the first statement
C   if the first statement is true but the second statement is false
D   if the first statement is false but the second statement is true
E   if both statements are false

Directions summarised:

A:	True	True	second statement is **a correct explanation** of the first
B:	True	True	second statement is **NOT a correct explanation** of the first
C:	True	False	
D:	False	True	
E:	False	False	

Q9

■   *Statement 1*: A community pharmacy that offers remuneration above
    the national average and is refitted to provide excellent working
    conditions will not necessarily improve the level of staff motivation.
■   *Statement 2*: The 'hygiene factors' identified by Herzberg can be
    demotivating if they are poor, but do not tend to be motivating if
    they are good.

Q10

■   *Statement 1*: A manager setting up a new community pharmacy team
    would ideally try and recruit team members with different strengths.
■   *Statement 2*: Belbin demonstrated that for a team to be balanced it
    should demonstrate a number of different roles linked to personality
    type.

Case studies

Level 1

Sheetal is part of a group of four final-year pharmacy undergraduates that are required to make a formal presentation on a clinical case study. The presentation forms part of their final assessment for a module. The groups have been allocated randomly and Sheetal is very concerned as she has not worked with any of the students in her group before. The first planning meeting did not go well as the group appears to be extremely diverse. She makes a mental note of the behaviour of her colleagues:

- Adil appears to be very loud and has many good ideas but is not very willing to listen to other viewpoints
- Angela is extremely quiet and does not contribute to the discussion but is known to be very reliable and hard working
- Liam is well known for achieving excellent academic results and has an excellent grasp of the case study. Unfortunately he comes across as arrogant and unwilling to co-operate with other members of the group
- Sheetal is a conscientious student and feels concerned that the group will not work well together and that this will have a negative impact on their assessment.

The group is due to meet again next week for another planning meeting.

- What advice would you give to Sheetal to ensure that the next meeting runs more smoothly and is more productive?

Level 2

Michelle has been asked by her preregistration tutor to organise a health-promotion activity in the pharmacy on National No Smoking Day. She is pleased to have been trusted with this event and her tutor has suggested that she should call a meeting of the dispensary team to discuss possible activities and plan the day.

- Produce a brief bullet-pointed list of constructive advice for Michelle on:
  - how she should plan the meeting
  - a suitable agenda for this meeting with proposed timing
  - how she should follow up the meeting.

Level 3

John has now been registered for 3 years and is due to be relocated to manage a pharmacy recently acquired by his employer.

The pharmacy is situated on the edge of a large market town. The business has been quite neglected and has been running on locums for the past year. On John's initial visit to the pharmacy he makes some notes of the major points related to this pharmacy:

- prescription items approximately 1000 per month
- retail turnover very low
- retail floor area large and 'empty' appearance. Good parking facilities
- appearance of store very dirty and neglected. The dispensary in particular looks very untidy and disorganised
- dispensary grossly overstocked
- there is no prescription-collection service
- staff:
  - one full-time supervisor, suffers from poor health and has had a lot of sick leave, attitude is quite negative particularly towards the employing organisation. The supervisor is not used to being managed or having a permanent manager and is not at all involved in the pharmacy as she sees this 'as the work of the pharmacist'
  - one part-time member of staff who works for three hours each morning, and appears to be very slow in her work and also very reluctant to become involved in the dispensary
  - Saturday staff: two young students – inexperienced but seem to be well motivated and keen to learn
- some loyal customers, but mainly passing trade
- the nearest pharmacy is on the same road and about 200 m away on a busy part of the road

- Carry out a SWOT (strengths, weaknesses, opportunities, threats) analysis of this business.
- What are John's priorities as a new manager? Construct a time chart of suggested actions for John during his first 2 months as a manager.

References

1   The Management Standards Centre website. www.management-standards.org.uk (accessed 4 September 2007).

2   Covey S. *The Seven Habits of Highly Effective People*. London: Simon and Schuster, 1989.

3   Calder G. Motivating pharmacists. *Pharm J* 2000; **264**: 729–731. www.pjonline.com/editorial/20000513/articles/motivating.html (accessed 7 September 2007).

4   Leigh A. *20 Ways to Manage Better*, 3rd edn. London: Chartered Institute of Personnel Development, 2001.

5   McGuire R. How to manage meetings effectively. *Pharm J* 2002; **268**: 766–767.

6   Walters M, ed. *The Performance Management Handbook*. London: Institute of Personnel and Development, 1995.

7   Department of Health. *Pharmacy in the Future*. London: The Stationery Office, 2000.
8   Department of Health. *Pharmacy Workforce in the New NHS: making the best use of staff to deliver the NHS pharmacy programme*. London: Department of Health, 2002.
9   Shaw ME. *Group Dynamics: the psychology of small group behaviour*, 3rd edn. New York: McGraw-Hill, 1981.
10   Katzenback JR, Smith DK. *The Wisdom of Teams; Creating the High Performance Organisation*. Boston: Harvard Business School Press, 1993.
11   Belbin Team Roles website. www.belbin.com/belbin-team-roles.htm (accessed 4 September 2007).
12   Wilson DA. Managing information (Institute of Management Foundation). Oxford: Butterworth Heinemann, in Association with the Institute of Management, 1993.
13   Blanchard K. *Leadership and the One Minute Manager*. London: Harper Collins, 1994.

Further information

Institute of Pharmacy Management website. www.ipmi.org.uk/ (accessed 4 September 2007).
McGuire R. How to build a successful team. *Pharm J* 2002; **269**: 814–816.

Training and development of the pharmacy team

Excellence is an art won by training and habituation. We do not act rightly because we have virtue or excellence, but we rather have those because we have acted rightly. We are what we repeatedly do. Excellence, then, is not an act but a habit.

(Aristotle)

Checkpoint

Before reading on, think about the following questions to identify your own knowledge gaps in this area:

- What formal qualifications are required for different types of pharmacy support staff?
- How would you carry out a training needs analysis in the pharmacy?
- Describe four different types of training method that could be used in a community pharmacy and the advantages and disadvantages of each method.
- How can training be evaluated?

At the outset it is important to differentiate between training and learning. Training is something that one person does to another. Learning is something that we can only do for ourselves. The community pharmacist is actively involved in the training of other members of the team. A logical starting point when considering the training and development of the pharmacy team is to consider who is being trained and for what purpose.

Pharmacy support team

The subject of skill mix in the delivery of healthcare has been actively debated in recent years. Optimising the mix of skills across the health sector is considered to be a viable way of meeting patient needs,

providing enhanced roles for staff and addressing recruitment and retention issues. Assessing and modifying skill mix in community pharmacy is
difficult because of the diverse and complex nature of community pharmacy.[1] A large study to explore and define the roles of dispensary support
staff looked at different community pharmacies and ways that support
staff operated.[2] The findings illustrate that the community pharmacy
environment is complex and diverse in terms of the roles played by
dispensary support staff. The study included the following different types
of pharmacy:

- a pharmacy where all support staff have distinct roles that do not overlap
- a pharmacy dominated by the owner-manager who is involved closely in
  the day-to-day activities
- a technician-led pharmacy that is highly efficient but the technician is
  unwilling to delegate tasks and decision making
- a pharmacy with a pharmacy technician that provides a highly focused
  dispensing service
- a team of support staff that have effectively run the pharmacy with a
  locum pharmacist in the absence of a permanent pharmacy manager
- a pharmacy that demonstrated a strong team spirit among the support
  staff to ensure that all tasks were completed.

The experienced community pharmacist may have experienced all of the
above different work scenarios and combinations of working patterns.
The variation across community pharmacies as well as the number, type
and activities of pharmacy staff must be considered in the development
of different models of skill mix.[3]

It is important to be clear at the outset what types of support staff
exist in the pharmacy, how their role is defined and what formal qualifications are required.

The *Medicines Ethics and Practice Guide* defines three main types of
support staff:[4]

- pharmacy technicians
- dispensing/pharmacy assistants
- medicine counter assistants.

Medicine counter assistants

Medicine counter assistants (MCAs) are given delegated authority by the
pharmacist under a medicines protocol to sell medicines. Since 1996 it
has been a requirement that any MCA should have undertaken or be
undertaking an accredited course relevant to their role in the sale of
medicines and provision of healthcare advice. The Royal Pharmaceutical
Society of Great Britain (RPSGB) requirement is that the course should
cover the knowledge and understanding associated with specific units of

the Scottish/National Vocational Qualification (S/NVQ) Level 2 in Pharmacy Services. The specified units are 2.04 and 2.05 which include the sale of over-the-counter medicines, prescription reception and issuing completed prescriptions. Full details of accredited courses and the specific knowledge and understanding required by the Pharmacy Services Level 2 units are available in the document *Training Requirements for Medicine Counter Assistants*.[5] MCAs are required to be enrolled on a suitable training programme within 3 months of working on the medicine counter, or as soon as is practical within local training arrangements. The training programme should be completed within a 3-year time period.

Dispensing/pharmacy assistants

Up to January 2005 there were no formal training requirements for members of staff working in the dispensary area either as a dispenser or pharmacy assistant. There was quite a lot of confusion over these titles as it covered a range of staff from the highly experienced and qualified pharmacy technician to a school leaver who is working in a dispensary and has limited experience. To try and clarify the situation for their own employees, many companies had already introduced their own internal training schemes at two levels: pharmacy assistant and dispenser. The pharmacy assistant carried out routine dispensing tasks under the supervision of a dispenser. The situation was further confused by use of other titles such as healthcare assistant and dispensing assistant.

Pharmacists have a professional obligation to ensure that dispensing and pharmacy assistants are competent in the areas in which they are working. This competency is defined by a minimum standard equivalent to the new Pharmacy Services S/NVQ Level 2 qualification or undertaking training towards this qualification. This requirement applies to staff working in the following areas:

- sale of over-the-counter medicines and the provision of information to customers on symptoms and products
- prescription receipt and collection
- the assembly of prescribed items (including the generation of labels)
- ordering, receiving and storing pharmaceutical stock
- the supply of pharmaceutical stock
- preparation for the manufacture of pharmaceutical products (including aseptic products)
- manufacture and assembly of medicinal products (including aseptic products).

The dispensing or pharmacy assistant should be enrolled on a training programme within 3 months of starting their new role or as soon as is practical within local training arrangements. The training programme must be completed within a 3-year time period and the type of training programme selected will depend on the specific job role of the member of staff. There are four acceptable training programmes:

- Pharmacy Services S/NVQ Level 2
- relevant units of Pharmacy Services S/NVQ Level 2
- a training programme accredited to be of an equivalent level to S/NVQ Level 2 (for example an accredited company training scheme)
- relevant units of a training programme accredited to be of an equivalent level to S/NVQ Level 2.

During the introduction of this requirement there was a grandparenting clause where existing staff were exempted by a statement of competence from their supervising pharmacist submitted to the RPSGB.

Pharmacy technician

A pharmacy technician is a person who holds a S/NVQ Pharmacy Services Level 3 qualification, or a qualification that has previously been recognised by employers as a valid qualification for pharmacy technicians. The pharmacy technician has a wide variety of skills in the supply and use of medicines, and this is often recognised by the formal management role they have in a pharmacy. The RPSGB opened a voluntary register of pharmacy technicians in January 2005 and issued guidelines for acceptable qualifications.[6] This means that the title 'pharmacy technician' will become protected in law and registration will be mandatory. There will be an initial transitional period during which grandparenting arrangements will apply to technicians who predate S/NVQ qualifications, who can provide evidence of alternative qualification and recent work experience as a pharmacy technician. Transitional grandparenting arrangements will only apply until 2 years after the introduction of statutory registration. A full list of qualifications that apply during this period is available on the RPSGB website.[5]

In addition to training MCAs, dispensers and pharmacy technicians, the pharmacist may also be involved in the training and development of:

- pharmacy technicians undertaking extended roles such as an accredited checking technician (ACT)
- preregistration pharmacy graduates
- undergraduate pharmacy students undertaking vacation employment.

Training and development in a community pharmacy can be a complex area, given the wide-ranging skill mix issues and the external training requirements for staff members undertaking different roles. The profile of the pharmacist as a training manager will be raised further, as new pharmacy services are implemented, more accredited checking technicians are introduced, and the issue of pharmacist supervision becomes less pre-scriptive. This chapter aims to provide an overview of important training issues to support the pharmacist in this expanding role.

Training needs analysis

Careful analysis of training needs is the foundation of all good training practice. Without a systematic training needs analysis, our training methods and use of resources become questionable. The first question to ask is: 'What is a training need?'

It is obvious that an experienced ACT may need, for example, to develop specific IT management skills, whereas a newly appointed MCA is more concerned with being able to operate a cash till. However the difference in the content of training requirements for different personnel is only a superficial insight into training needs analysis (TNA).

TNA is concerned with the following areas:

- types of learning need
- organisational needs
- individual needs
- key task analysis
- competency analysis.

There have been many attempts to classify types of learning. Bloom's Taxonomy of Learning proposes that there are four types of learning:[7]

- cognitive (thinking and analysing)
- affective (feelings and attitudes)
- psychomotor (physical)
- interpersonal (relationships with people).

Theoretical classifications may seem artificial in practical workplace situations as there is a certain amount of overlap. The advantage of looking at learning needs in more detail is that the training manager starts to plan the training programme around a specific need rather than using the approach that one size fits all approach. (See Example 3.1 overleaf.)

The needs of the organisation also need to be entered into the TNA equation to achieve a positive outcome. For the employee pharmacist this may involve looking at the wider corporate picture. The self-employed pharmacist will take time to reflect on personal business priorities.

To facilitate this process it is useful to ask questions such as:

- what business objectives have the highest priority over the next 12 months?
- how successful is the organisation engaging with the contractual framework for community pharmacy?

Example 3.1

Mark is a pharmacy technician who has excellent theoretical knowledge and performs well in operating an efficient dispensing service. However, his interpersonal skills and attitude towards customers and colleagues is a constant source of concern. Should this member of the team be required to complete more distance learning training packages and theoretical learning, when his real learning needs have not been addressed? Community pharmacy can provide many examples where the type of learning need for individuals has not been considered fully.

- are there any new plans for offering new innovative services or offering different product ranges?
- is there any new legislation that may affect the way the team operates?
- are there any plans for physical changes to premises or upgrading of information technology systems?

Often when broader questions are considered there can be seen to be some common ground and this will provide a different organisational perspective to the overall training plan.

Another important component of TNA is the consideration of individual learning needs. The goals and aspirations of pharmacy employees are likely to differ from those of the organisation. For example the competent dispensing assistant may have goals that include working for a different employer and at a higher level. This excellent team member may want to become a registered pharmacy technician and work for a large multiple. The unspoken individual agenda may often be due to the employer not being willing to invest in highly transferable skills, and subsequently losing a highly valuable member of their team. When looking at individual goals, open communication is vital to establish how the employee feels about their own job role. For example the pharmacist may perceive that their pharmacy technician could work more quickly and process prescription items with greater efficiency. The pharmacy technician may have the view that the patient medication record (PMR) system is outdated and the number of support staff is not adequate for the level of business. It is only by open and honest communication that you can establish if there is a training need or if the deficiency is caused by other factors that are unrelated to training. The consideration of individual learning needs is vital if a realistic training programme is to be implemented.

The next stage of the TNA process is to analyse job roles and key tasks in the pharmacy. There are different approaches to this task and a better result is obtained if information is gathered from a variety of sources. Questions that could be asked include:

- what is the expectation of each job role from the pharmacy manager?
- how does the job holder see their role and responsibilities?
- is there any evidence from diary keeping or work shadowing? This information would need to be used to assess the details of what a job entails over a period of several weeks.
- is there any information from team meetings or discussions with work colleagues about how different members of the team perceive different tasks?
- what documentation is available on job descriptions and key outputs?

Having obtained a clearer view of what each role entails in your pharmacy, the next stage is to break down each job into key tasks according to what knowledge, skills and attitudes are required.

For example the MCA may have the following key tasks:

- merchandising medicines
- medicines stock control and management
- sale of medicines
- answering general customer queries and acting as a receptionist
- prescription reception
- store housekeeping duties.

By looking at the knowledge, skills and attitudes that are required by each key task, a general picture should start to emerge. It may be for example that the experienced counter assistant needs to develop more advanced customer care skills and be able to act as a receptionist for the running of a pharmacy-based weight-management clinic. The time and training required to achieve this objective may mean that some non-customer-based tasks will need to be relinquished to other members of the team. In this scenario, the range of key skills required by this member of staff will shift, and this needs to be acknowledged in the planning of training. A community pharmacist interested in the training and development of staff should aim to produce a matrix of all the job roles in the business and the key skills required. Provided this information is regularly updated, it will prove invaluable in ensuring that training is relevant to the needs of the staff and ultimately the business.

A more recent approach to TNA is the concept of competence. The competence-based approach looks more closely at the behaviour that results from specific knowledge, skills and attitudes. Competency is defined as being able to perform 'whole' work roles to the standards expected in employment and real working environments.[8] There are two main approaches when using competence as a means of identifying learning needs: input approaches and the outcomes model.

The input approach focuses on the blend of skills, personal attributes and attitudes that enable people to perform effectively in the workplace. This is all about patterns of behaviour that employees need to bring with them to do a job effectively. The outcomes approach is the model on which the NVQ system is based, where the employee is matched against a set of performance standards. The use of performance indicators is critical when using a competence-based approach. It will involve asking questions such as:

- what does good look like?
- what is acceptable?
- what is poor?

In pharmacy practice the competence-based approach is widely used and forms the basis of the preregistration training programme. The use of a specific template of competencies gives the pharmacy graduate a clear idea of where they are heading, and is a valuable tool in determining their own training needs.

Successful TNA involves adopting a reflective approach and looking at the pharmacy with a critical eye. What is certain is that the time spent on this vital process of assessing training needs is never wasted.

Training methods in the pharmacy

Having established specific training needs, the next stage is to determine what training methods are most appropriate. Some of the factors to be considered when selecting or designing the most appropriate training method are summarised in Figure 3.1.

The pharmacy manager will need to consider such factors as:

- time resources available and ensuring that adequate time for training is built into the working week
- cost as part of the overall training budget
- organisational constraints such as how the training will complement the existing company training plan
- strengths and weaknesses of the pharmacist or staff member delivering the training
- the physical work environment, as this will also have some influence on the training methods used. For example there is much more flexibility if there is a designated training room that is well equipped for both individual and group training. This facility is only likely to exist in a large pharmacy and the pharmacist working in a smaller pharmacy will need to look carefully at how space and physical resources can be used to

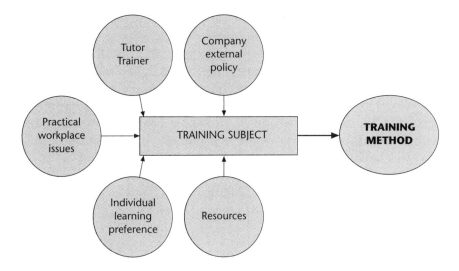

Figure 3.1 Factors that influence the choice of training method in the pharmacy.

facilitate training. It is inappropriate to expect members of the pharmacy team to study distance learning material while on the shop floor
■ preferred learning methods for individual members of staff, which will also influence the type of training method selected. Some members of staff will prefer a more active approach to learning and gain more from being allowed to explore, test and learn by doing. Others prefer a more passive approach and will gain more by observing, questioning, interpreting and reviewing activities. Other members of the team will prefer to learn in a group situation and reflect ideas off their colleagues.

There are three broad categories of training method:

■ trainer-centred training
■ learner-centred training
■ coaching.

Trainer-centred training includes any type of training where the trainer controls the pace and content of learning. This will include formal presentations and demonstrations, either to an individual or a group. The learner may slow the training down by asking a lot of questions but the pace is ultimately set by the trainer. Role-plays and practical exercises are also trainer centred as the trainer sets the training content and draws out the key learning points.

Learner-centred training is at the opposite end of the spectrum and is designed to give the learner complete control over their learning. The established methods of learner-centred training include the use of printed training materials, books, journals and self-study materials. Learner-centred training can be made more active by the use of self-development questionnaires and personal learning logs. Increasingly learner-centred learning uses information and learning technology such as DVD and CD-ROM packages or internet based e-learning resources.

Coaching is a method of training that allows trainer and learner to develop a learning partnership and to share control. This method of training is particularly appropriate to community pharmacy and will be discussed later in this chapter.

Many community pharmacies use a combination of distance learning programmes and on-the-job training to develop their support staff.

The main training methods used in the pharmacy are summarised in Figure 3.2.

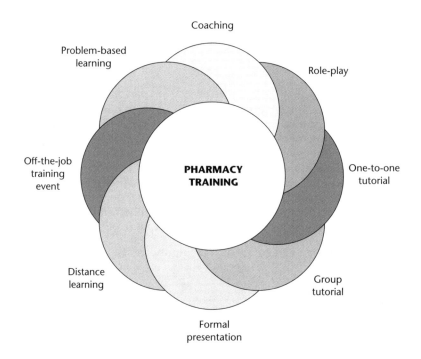

Figure 3.2 Types of training in the community pharmacy.

On-the-job training

Successful on-the-job training involves:

- a clear identification of the level of support that is needed
- a clear identification of the most suitable person to give this support.

The traditional approach to training a new member of staff is to ask a more experienced member of staff to oversee their work and provide on-the-job training on an informal basis. This traditional 'sit next to Nelly' approach clearly has disadvantages, in particular the duplication of any poor working practices that an experienced employee may have developed over a number of years. On-the-job learning needs to be carefully planned for it to be fully effective. It may involve a formal 'buddy system' with regular reviews and a clear competence-based framework that can be assessed at regular intervals. Alternatively it may involve working through the various elements of a task in a logical sequence with different coaches for each stage of the task (Table 3.1).

Table 3.1 Examples of on-the-job training and identification of a suitable coach for a new dispensing assistant

Task	Coach
Prescription reception procedure	Experienced counter assistant
Handing out prescriptions	Pharmacist or pharmacy technician
Dealing with the initial stages of a customer complaint	Pharmacist or pharmacy technician
Putting away stock in the dispensary	Dispensing assistant

In community pharmacy where there is often the question of patient safety it can be inappropriate to let the new trainee work through problems on their own and much of the early training will be working through common standard operating procedures (SOPs). However, there is a place for allowing the trainee to tackle certain tasks with little input or supervision, provided this is followed up with a detailed discussion and review of how they approached the task. Learning by doing is a powerful training tool as long as it is followed up with supportive feedback. For example the new MCA will sometimes have to interact with difficult and demanding customers. It is important that the new team member has adequate opportunity to discuss their experience of dealing with customers with a more experienced member of staff. When planning on-the-job training there should be a clear distinction between tasks that have a clear SOP and tasks where a certain amount of initiative and flexibility are required.

On-the-job training checklist

The following questions provide a useful checklist for on the job pharmacy training:

- is the training programme properly planned? (Check for natural progression within the programme from simple to more complex tasks)
- is there the time and resources to ensure that the trainee is adequately supported? (A weekly meeting needs to be scheduled to discuss progress and offer the opportunity for communication)
- is there a system of documentation that is transparent and allows the trainee and the trainer to monitor progress? It is vital that all training is clearly documented to prove that training has taken place
- is there an effective coach available to deliver the training? When selecting a coach consider the level of skill required and choose a member of the team who is able to offer full support through the training process.
- have any health and safety hazards been taken into account?
- how will competence be measured?
- how will the training be evaluated?

The two main benefits of on-the-job learning in the pharmacy include:

- training is immediately seen as relevant to the job as it is carried out in a real workplace setting.
- training is provided at a time that is relevant and fits in with the immediate needs of the trainee. This is in contrast to off-the-job training, as the training may be appropriate when planned but sometimes loses its relevance as the trainee becomes more experienced.

Off-the-job training

Off-the-job learning such as training days or regular day-release courses can be a useful way of providing background information. Many employees are interested in completing a recognised course such as a BTEC/NVQ course delivered by a further education institution.

A number of issues need to be considered before enrolling members of staff on to externally delivered courses:

- is the course relevant to the training needs of the employee?
- will the course include work-based exercises? How relevant will the exercises be to the pharmacy?
- is there sufficient time available to attend the course and complete all required coursework and study?

- how will the absence of the employee from the workplace be covered?
- what are the financial implications for this type of training? Costs to be considered should include course fees and associated costs (for example travel costs and exam fees) and the cost of staff absence from the pharmacy. The high cost of this type of training will also mean that the retention of staff trained by this cost-intensive method will need to be considered.

Distance learning

Distance learning by means of workbooks, training manuals and inter-active e-learning are commonly used training methods to train pharmacy support staff. The main advantages of distance learning are flexibility and cost-effectiveness. The disadvantage of this type of training method is that a high level of individual motivation is required. Distance learning courses that are well supported and supplemented by structured on-the-job training are often the training method of choice in community pharmacy.

Making a presentation

This traditional training method is often impractical during working hours in a community pharmacy as it is not possible to release a number of people at any one time. However, this method is increasingly used out of normal working hours to communicate important information and offer supplementary training on topical or important areas. For example this training method may be chosen to train the team on a new POM (prescription only medicine) to P (pharmacy medicine) switch or to explain the service specification and SOPs for the delivery of a new pro-fessional service. If the presentation takes place outside working hours, there is a cost implication in terms of overtime payments for staff. The advantage of making a presentation is that a common message is deliv-ered to all staff members at the same time.

Sufficient thought needs to be given to the timing of a presentation. This will depend on local circumstances, working patterns and individual preferences. For example, some pharmacies have introduced successful breakfast training meetings. In other situations a meeting in the evening that includes a meal have proved popular. In view of the high cost of this type of training it is particularly important to be aware of the key factors that ensure a successful presentation. The old adage 'Fail to prepare, prepare to fail' is especially pertinent when it comes to delivering a pre-sentation. The presentation skills developed to train pharmacy staff will also be invaluable when a pharmacist is required to present a new service proposal to a local medical practice or primary care organisation.

The traditional approach to a presentation can be very effective:

- tell them what you are going to tell them
- tell them
- tell them what you have told them.

The structure of the presentation is made clear at the start. The content is delivered in a way that is appropriate for the audience and engages their interest and attention.

The key points are summarised at the end of the presentation to ensure that the right message has been conveyed.

Top tips for effective presentations

- The material needs to be structured in a logical way. It is important that there is a framework for the listener to relate to. During the preparation of the presentation it may take several attempts to obtain the best structure. This may be achieved by brainstorming with a small group of other people who are not connected with the presentation or some presenters prefer to use 'post it' notes that can be moved around several times until the preferred final format emerges.
- Be clear at the start of the presentation about your policy on questions. When will you ask questions? Questions may be asked at the beginning to check preliminary knowledge and understanding, during the presentation to ensure attention, or at the end to evaluate the understanding of the audience. When would you prefer to take questions from the audience? There may be a preference for a formal question and answer session at the end of the presentation, or you may prefer to allow questions at any time throughout the presentation.
- The most effective presentations are clearly set out and the audience has a clear idea of where the presentation is going and what to expect. For example in the introduction you could explain the structure of your presentation, what you hope to achieve in each section and how long each section will take.
- Signpost your presentation so that the audience is guided through the structure. This may involve using regular summaries so that learning is consolidated.
- Rehearse the presentation to ensure that the timing is correct and also ask a friend to point out any weak points such as areas where there is a lack of pace or the content needs further clarification.
- Be prepared for the unexpected. Think about the possibility of questions taking longer than anticipated, a technical hitch with your equipment or a confrontational audience member. A few

$\rightarrow$

minutes spent thinking about the 'What if?' scenarios and possible solutions will increase your confidence.

■ Cultivate a clear and pleasant speaking voice that is neither over-the-top enthusiastic or deadpan boring. From a listener's perspective it is easier to listen to a speaker who naturally modulates and varies in pace and emphasis.

■ Ask a close friend about any distracting physical or verbal mannerisms that you may have, as these may act as a barrier. Try to develop ways of removing these possible distractions.

■ Think about the perspective of the audience and try to gain as much rapport as possible by maintaining good eye contact, but not with individuals for a prolonged period as this will cause discomfort. Develop a scanning approach where you aim to engage individuals, and systematically scan different areas of the room to ensure that all listeners feel included.

■ Develop questioning skills that will provide you with information on how the audience understands the content of the presentation. It is useful to ask structured questions as the presentation progresses.

■ Use a variety and combination of visual aids to add interest to the presentation. The regular use of PowerPoint projection can become stale and the use of different interactive methods such as flip charts, white boards and 'post it' notes may add interest to the overall subject content.

Many managers can be fearful of making a presentation. In reality, many of the fears can be overcome by meticulous and careful planning. The presentation remains a powerful training tool that allows a direct and personal input into the development of a pharmacy team.

Using role-play

In any customer-focused business, role-play can be a useful training method. In a community pharmacy the use of role-play in the training of the pharmacy team can be applied to the following situations:

■ improving counselling skills and interaction with customers
■ developing teamwork, co-operation with colleagues and creative problem solving
■ improving listening skills with both customers and colleagues.

The overall aim of role-playing is to ask someone to play a role other than his or her own. This enables the team member to see the workplace through different eyes.

Examples 3.2

- It is valuable for a MCA to see the viewpoint of a customer who has a complaint and has been treated in a dismissive way. Taking on the role of the customer being shabbily treated helps to reinforce some of the tension and anxiety that the customer may experience.
- A pharmacy technician with new responsibility for managing different members of staff may find it beneficial to take on the role of being managed. A more experienced staff member plays the role of the pharmacy technician and uses examples of aggressive, passive and assertive management to provide the opportunity to explore methods of communication. The role reversal of the pharmacy technician who is put on the spot by their 'manager' offers the possibility of seeing examples of good and less-desirable management traits.

Many people are apprehensive about this training method and can dismiss this type of training as simple play acting and of no relevance. To gain maximum benefit from this method the role-play exercises must follow certain rules (see Top tips for role-playing exercises).

Top tips for role-playing exercises

- Be clear about exactly which competencies are trying to be developed. (Example: a role-play to demonstrate the importance of dealing with an aggressive customer in a calm manner.)
- Make sure the scenario is real and relevant to the workplace. (Keep a diary of real-life problems posed by customers or team members and take steps to use these as a training exercise at a later date, with some minor changes to preserve the anonymity of those involved.)
- Keep the role-play simple. The role-play characters may not have all the same information but the scenario should hang together as a whole. Avoid complicated plots and make it simple for the participants to carry out their role without being too worried about the details of the scenario.
- Prepare carefully for the role-play and allow sufficient time for constructive feedback and discussion.
- The partners in a role-play situation should be carefully matched to ensure that they will work well together and gain as much as possible from the experience.
- When providing feedback it is important to concentrate on the key player and the skills that are being developed in that participant. The key player should be asked to talk through their experience

$\rightarrow$

and the good and bad points of the role-play. This should be done before any of the other participants are invited to comment.

- Concentrate any discussion on behaviours and not on the person carrying out the role. In some cases it may be more appropriate to prepare a structured report form for all involved in the role-play, including any observers. This can act as a positive example on how to focus on the observed behaviours rather than on the personality of the team members involved.

If the initial barrier of awkward self-consciousness can be overcome, the use of role-play can be a powerful training tool to improve communication skills in the pharmacy. The difficulties and objections encountered in this type of training can seem trivial compared to the potentially enormous cost of poor communication with 'real' customers.

Group work

Group work may be useful when several members of staff are using a distance learning course and need clarification and extra input to certain areas of the course. For example, the pharmacist may decide to run a small-group session on controlled drugs for their trainee dispensing assistants. Many group training sessions revolve around a structured discussion followed by feedback. This may be a quick informal sharing of ideas and/ or may be a formal presentation to the rest of the group. Successful small-group training is dependent on certain key practical principles (see Top tips for successful group training sessions below).

Coaching skills

In a busy community pharmacy, coaching is a practical training method that avoids some of the disadvantages of other training methods. Coaching involves the pharmacist asking questions and listening to the replies in order to gauge what the level of their input should be. With coaching the learner is totally involved in setting goals and answering informal questions. This means that both coach and learner are encouraged by each other's involvement in the process. Coaching can be applied to both individuals and the whole team.

One useful approach to coaching is the GROW model. GROW is an acronym for:

Top tips for successful group training sessions

- Be clear about the learning objectives for the session and the format of the available time for the session. Where possible involve group members in the formulation of learning outcomes.
- Encourage the group to take on different roles such as chairperson, scribe, presenter or researcher. The group members will need to be reminded to change roles during the next session.
- Be clear about the practical details such as the length of the session, the format of the feedback session and what materials are available.
- If necessary the trainer may need to guide the discussion back on track with a few questions, but avoiding the pitfall of joining in the group discussion.
- In a community pharmacy setting the group members will be used to working with one another. If there is a new member of staff or a visiting participant (for example from another pharmacy), the trainer should take some time to ensure that all members are introduced. If the group is new to this type of work then time should also be spent establishing ground rules for group working.

- goal
- (current) reality
- options
- will.

Using these four stages, a coach can structure a useful coaching session. A coaching session does not need to be formal and scheduled into the working week. Effective coaching is often spontaneous and designed to respond to practical workplace training needs.

The model uses the following stages:

1 establish the goal
2 examine current reality
3 explore the options
4 establish the will.

Establish the goal

The pharmacist with their team member defines and agrees the goal to be achieved using SMART (specific, measurable, achievable, relevant and timed) objectives as discussed in Chapter 1. (See Examples 3.3 below.)

Successful coaching requires a clearly defined outcome at the outset, before moving on to the next stage.

Examples 3.3

- *Medicine counter assistant*: to be able to recognise the symptoms of conjunctivitis and know when the recommendation of chloramphenicol eye drops is appropriate and also know when to refer to the pharmacist.
- *Dispensing assistant*: to be able to measure a patient for compression hosiery correctly and order the appropriate product.
- *Pharmacy technician*: to be able to set up a supply service to a newly acquired residential home.
- *Preregistration graduate*: to be able to conduct a patient interview as part of a project to produce pharmaceutical care plans.

For all of these examples the pharmacist will need to ask questions at the outset about how the team member will know when they have achieved their goal, for example questions such as:

- how will you know that you are competent to supply choramphenicol eye drops?
- how will you be able to determine that you can accurately measure for compression hosiery and supply the correct product?
- how will you prove that the residential home is fully set up and all paperwork and patient medication record (PMR) systems are fully operational for the first month of supply?
- What criteria will you use to determine how successful you are at interviewing a patient?

Examine current reality

During this stage of the coaching process the pharmacy team member should be asked in some detail about their current reality. This is an important stage and involves an honest approach to the situation as it stands. For example the pharmacy technician may have very limited experience of working with residential homes and need a lot of direction to set up the necessary records. Alternatively the pharmacy technician may have wide experience of working with residential homes but not have been involved in the initial setting-up stage before. The aim of this part of the coaching session is to ask searching questions that enable both the team member and the pharmacist coach to assess current reality.

Explore the options

Having made a realistic assessment of where the team member is in terms of solving their problem, the next stage is to explore the options available to solve the problem and discuss the positive and negative aspects of each option. It is important that the team member comes up with most of the suggestions. For example the MCA may suggest:

■ completion of a distance learning package on conjunctivitis and chloramphenicol eye drops
■ job shadowing a more experienced MCA when they make a sale of chloramphenicol drops
■ a tutorial session with the pharmacist to ensure that the assistant has sufficient background knowledge.

It is useful for the pharmacist at this stage to ask leading questions to ensure that the most appropriate options are selected. Typical questions could include:

■ what else could you do?
■ are there any difficulties with job shadowing and how could these be overcome?

Establish the will

This fourth and final stage is all about asking the team member to commit to a specific course of action. As the team member has already identified the goal, looked at where they stand in terms of achieving this goal and also explored possible options, they are in a strong position to specify how they are going to progress towards their goal. For example the pharmacist will ask the MCA how they intend to complete the distance learning package or observe more experienced colleagues. Again, this stage is marked by leading questions from the coach such as:

■ what do you intend to do . . . and when?
■ how will you overcome any problems with this course of action?
■ what else will you be doing?

Coaching is a skill that is invaluable in the community pharmacy setting. This well-established training tool is dependent on the pharmacist habitually asking leading open questions, listening attentively to the response and facilitating the ongoing development of both individuals and the team.

Evaluation of training

The evaluation of training has three main purposes:[9]

■ it provides feedback to the trainer in terms of the extent to which the

training objectives were met, and provides some information on particular learning activities. Did the training meet its objectives?
■ it offers a control process and allows the manager to assess if the training delivered fits in with the goals of the wider organisation. Did the training make a difference to the wider organisation?
■ the opportunity for intervention as the manager is involved in the total training process by considering training both before and after the programme has been delivered. Was the training good value for money?

The manager should be aware of the following areas:

■ ineffective training is not only a waste of time and money it is also very demotivating for employees and will make the trainee less likely to engage positively with future training programmes
■ there has to be a strong link between training and the overall performance of the organisation
■ in view of the high cost of training, any training investment will need to be justified.

Levels of training evaluation

There are different levels of training evaluation as outlined in Figure 3.3.

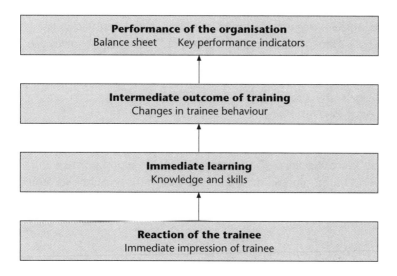

Figure 3.3 Different levels of training evaluation.

The different levels of training evaluation include the stages below:

■ *the reactions of the trainees*: this is sometimes referred to as the 'happy sheet' as the focus tends to be on the immediate impression of the trainee such as the quality of refreshments and clarity of visual aids rather than the impact of the training on their working practice

- *the immediate learning that has taken place*: this is the immediate impression of the trainee in terms of what they feel they have gained from the programme
- *the intermediate outcome of the training*: this evaluation focuses on the change in behaviour of the employee and their approach to their working practice
- *the ultimate outcome*: this is the effect of the training on the performance of the organisation and is usually measured by looking at a balance sheet rather than the behaviour of an individual.

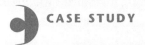 **CASE STUDY**

Case study 3.1: evaluation

Julie is an experienced pharmacy technician who was recommended by her manager to attend a one-day training course. The course was aimed at technicians providing support to pharmacists interested in launching a weight-management service to patients. The service involves the provision of orlistat to suitable patients through a patient group direction (PGD).

Training evaluation

Reactions of the trainee

Julie enjoyed the one-day course and thought the venue and refreshments were excellent. The practical session on blood pressure monitoring and blood glucose measurement was 'rather rushed' according to the feedback sheet, and her impression was that the 'trainer assumed too much prior knowledge'.

The immediate outcome

The pharmacist discussed the training day with the technician and asked some leading questions about the content of the day and her understanding of the weight-management programme. The pharmacist noted that the technician had a good knowledge of the programme and offered to supplement the practical session with some practice blood pressure and blood glucose measurements.

→

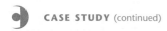 **CASE STUDY** (continued)

The intermediate outcome

The technician started to work towards a launch date for the new service and worked with the pharmacist to achieve competence in the various stages of managing the programme.

The ultimate outcome

After three months of offering the service the pharmacy manager noted the number of clients that had taken up this service and the profit generated by each PGD sale. The pharmacist manager looked at the time taken by the technician and pharmacist and took these costs into account. The conclusion was that the first 3 months had been highly successful and the projected figures looked promising.

The initial reactions of the technician were not completely positive and it appears that a substantial amount of tutorial work was done by the pharmacist subsequent to the training day. There is some doubt about the value of the training day and if this type of training event was necessary in this case. The overall ultimate outcome of the training provided by the pharmacist appears to have been very positive.

The community pharmacy manager will use different training providers and approaches to training. It is vital that all training in the pharmacy is evaluated at different levels to ensure that the training provision meets the needs of the business.

Implications for practice

Activity 1

Consider each member of your pharmacy team and perform a training needs analysis (TNA) of your pharmacy. Present your observations in the following format:

- types of learning need
- organisational needs
- individual needs
- key task analysis
- competency analysis.

How does your TNA differ from the reality of what is taking place?

Activity 2

Select a recent POM to P switch and plan a training event on this product area.

- Plan the event carefully ensuring that it is at a suitable level.
- Deliver and evaluate the training at different levels.

Multiple choice questions

Directions for questions 1 and 2: each of the questions or incomplete statements in this section is followed by five suggested answers. Select the best answer in each case.

Q1 Bloom's taxonomy of learning proposes all of the following types of learning *except*:

A Cognitive
B Reactive
C Affective
D Psychomotor
E Interpersonal

Q2 Training needs analysis is concerned with all of the following areas *except*:

A Organisational priorities
B Trainer competence
C Individual trainee competence
D Key task analysis
E Types of learning need

Directions for questions 3 to 5: for each numbered question select the one lettered option above it which is most closely related to it. Within each group of questions each lettered option may be used once, more than once, or not at all.

A Coaching
B Role-play
C Distance learning
D Competence based
E Presentation

Select from A to E which one of the above fits the following statements:

Q3 The GROW model can be used for this training method.
Q4 This informal type of training can be unscheduled and requires a good working relationship with the trainee.

Q5   A trainer-centred training method.

Directions for questions 6 to 8: each of the questions or incomplete statements in this section is followed by three responses. For each question ONE or MORE of the responses is (are) correct. Decide which of the responses is (are) correct. Then choose:

A   if **1**, **2** and **3** are correct
B   if **1** and **2** only are correct
C   if **2** and **3** only are correct
D   if **1** only is correct
E   if **3** only is correct

Directions summarised:
A: 1, 2, 3   B: 1, 2 only   C: 2, 3 only   D: 1 only   E: 3 only

Q6   Which of the following statements about medicine counter assistants (MCAs) is (are) correct?

1   It is a requirement that any MCA should have undertaken or be undertaking an accredited course relevant to their role.
2   MCAs are allowed up to 6 months before enrolling on an accredited course.
3   There is no time limit for the completion of an accredited training course for MCAs.

Q7   Which of the following statements about dispensing assistants is (are) correct?

1   The competency of a dispensing or pharmacy assistant is defined by the minimum of a S/NVQ Level 2 qualification, or undertaking training towards this qualification.
2   A company training scheme for pharmacy assistants would need to be accredited.
3   The competency requirement of a dispensing or pharmacy assistant does *not* apply if the assistant is only involved in the ordering, receiving and storing of pharmaceutical stock.

Q8   Which of the following statements about pharmacy technicians is (are) correct?

1   The title of pharmacy technician will become protected in law.
2   An NVQ qualification in pharmacy services (Level 3) is a recognisable qualification for a pharmacy technician.
3   Pharmacy technicians who do not have NVQ qualifications are not eligible for registration with the RPSGB.

Directions for questions 9 and 10: The following questions consist of a statement in the left-hand column followed by a second statement in the right-hand column.

Decide whether the first statement is true or false.

Decide whether the second statement is true or false.

Then choose:

A   if both statements are true and the second statement is a correct explanation of the first statement
B   if both statements are true but the second statement is NOT a correct explanation of the first statement
C   if the first statement is true but the second statement is false
D   if the first statement is false but the second statement is true
E   if both statements are false

Directions summarised:

A:	True	True	second statement is **a correct explanation** of the first
B:	True	True	second statement is **NOT a correct explanation** of the first
C:	True	False	
D:	False	True	
E:	False	False	

Q9

- *Statement 1*: When assessing an MCA on the ability to receive prescriptions, the pharmacist will refer to the SOP for this process and also examples of good, acceptable and poor practice in this area.
- *Statement 2*: The use of performance indicators is critical when using a competence-based training approach.

Q10

- *Statement 1*: The most important evaluation of any training is feedback from the trainee on what they feel they have gained from the training programme.
- *Statement 2*: Training evaluation should be carried out at a number of different levels.

Case studies

Level 1

A group of third-year pharmacy undergraduates is asked to assess a 15 minute presentation by their colleagues. Before the presentation, their tutor would like the group to have some ownership over the marking scheme for this piece of assessed work. The tutor invites suggestions from all members of the group and intends to use a compilation of these suggestions to produce a summary mark scheme.

- Make a list of criteria that you would suggest for inclusion in a marking scheme for a presentation.

Level 2

Kerry is a preregistration trainee in a large community pharmacy. The pharmacy has a very intensive medicine counter business which is managed by three able and experienced MCAs. In the next month one of the counter assistants is moving to the dispensary area to start their training as a dispensing assistant. Two new part-time members of staff have been appointed to work on the medicines counter. Both new members of staff are experienced in working in a retail setting, but neither has experience of working in a pharmacy. Kerry's tutor has explained that she will ensure they are registered on a distance learning MCA course and has asked Kerry to organise some additional training sessions. As a starting point Kerry's tutor has suggested that she arranges a session on the sale of cough medicines.

- Kerry is asked to produce an outline plan of a 30-minute training session on this product area.
- What specific preregistration performance standards relate to this activity?

Level 3

Marie Logan has recently been appointed as the temporary pharmacy manager of a medium-sized pharmacy of a large multiple. The pharmacy is based on the edge of the town and is within easy access of several medical centres. There have been a number of staff training problems in this pharmacy and Marie has been appointed on a temporary basis to try and improve this area.

Marie makes the following observations about the pharmacy staff:

- Lorna is an MCA who is struggling to find time to complete the distance learning package that she started a year ago. She appears keen and is excellent with customers
- Beth is an MCA who has completed the distance learning package but still requires a lot of supervision. Marie has some concerns over the quality of advice that she is providing for customers
- Dan is at the local sixth form college and works evenings and Saturdays. He is employed on the medicine counter but is keen to become involved

in dispensary activities. He has completed the MCA course and has a
positive approach to his job
- Jeanne qualified as a dispenser several years ago and shows very little
interest in any additional training as she says that she is always too busy
- Jeanne is assisted by Sharon who is a school leaver and is a trainee
dispenser, but her progress has been rather slow on the course
- there is a very intensive supply service to 20 large residential care homes
that is well managed by Sandy who is a qualified pharmacy technician.
Sandy appears to be quite frustrated as she is finding the demands of the
care homes are increasing and feels quite isolated as she works away from
the main dispensing area
- there is a vacancy for a trainee dispenser but this has not yet been
advertised.

- Marie has been asked by her area manager to produce a proposed
training plan for this pharmacy, what should she include?

References

1   Hassell K, Shann P, Noyce P The complexities of skill mix in community
pharmacy. *Pharm J* 2002; **269**: 851–854.
2   Mullen R. *Skill Mix in Community Pharmacy: exploring and defining the
roles of dispensary support staff.* London: Royal Pharmaceutical Society of
Great Britain, 2004. www.pharmacy.manchester.ac.uk/cpws/publica-
tions/Reports/skillmix.pdf (accessed 4 September 2007).
3   Mullen R, Phul S, Cantrill J. Countdown to January 2005: standard operating procedures, regulation, training and skill mix issues for community pharmacy staff. *Int J Pharm Pract* 2003; **11**: R27.
4   Royal Pharmaceutical Society of Great Britain. *Medicines Ethics and
Practice. A guide for pharmacists and pharmacy technicians.* London: Royal
Pharmaceutical Society of Great Britain, 2007.
5   Royal Pharmaceutical Society of Great Britain. *Training Requirements for
Medicine Counter Assistants.* (Revised April 2007) www.rpsgb.org/pdfs/
medcountassiscourses.pdf (accessed 4 September 2007).
6   Royal Pharmaceutical Society of Great Britain. *Minimum Competence
Requirements and Pharmacy Technician Registration. Which policy applies to
me?* (May 2006) www.rpsgb.org/pdfs/techregdpaclarif.pdf (accessed 4
September 2007).
7   Atherton JS. Learning and Teaching: Bloom's Taxonomy. www.learning
andteaching.info/learning/bloomtax.htm (accessed 4 September 2007).
8   College of Pharmacy Practice. Competency and the extended role of the
pharmacy support staff. *Pharm J* 2000; **265**: 103–104.
9   Bramley P. *Evaluating Training*, 2nd edn. London: Chartered Institute of
Personnel and Development, 2003.

4

Contractual framework for community pharmacy

This is probably the most significant turning point for the NHS and for community pharmacy in the history of NHS pharmacy services.
(Rosie Winterton, Health Minister – Pharmaceutical Services Negotiating Committee (PSNC) conference on the new community pharmacy contract)

Checkpoint

Before reading on, think about the following questions to identify your own knowledge gaps in this area:

- What is the overall structure of the national contractual framework for community pharmacy?
- How is the contract monitored?
- What are the implications of the Disability Discrimination Act 1995 for community pharmacists?
- What is the general structure of a standard operating procedure?

The main focus of this chapter is on the provision of essential services as these must be provided by all community pharmacists in England and Wales. Some of the terminology used in Wales is different, such as the use of health boards, but the overall principles of the contract are the same. The arrangements for Scotland are different, and a brief overview of the Scottish contract is outlined at the end of this chapter. The chapter also includes sections on standard operating procedures, monitoring of the new contract and support for people with disabilities.

The main aims of the new contractual framework for community pharmacy are to:

- provide a set of minimum standards that reflect the needs of *Pharmacy in the Future: implementing the NHS Plan*[1]
- provide a reward system that recognises high-quality services and promotes best value for money
- utilise the skills of community pharmacists and their support staff and encourage the development of community services and integrated working.

In 2003, the PSNC, Department of Health and the NHS Confederation started negotiations for the new contractual framework for community pharmacy. The new national contract for community pharmacy in England and Wales was introduced in April 2005. The new contract aims to enable community pharmacies to contribute to NHS service provision for patients in four main areas:

- self-care
- management of long-term conditions
- public health
- improving access to services.

These priority areas are specified in the Department of Health's *Public Service Agreement.*[2]

Contract overview

An overview of the structure of the new contract for community pharmacy is provided in Figure 4.1. Pharmacy services are divided into three categories: essential, advanced and enhanced.

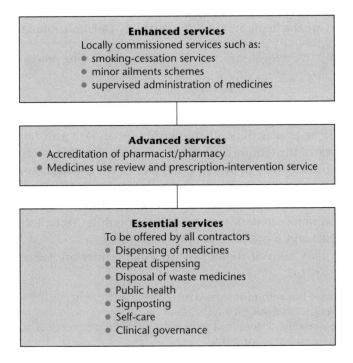

Figure 4.1 Contractual framework for community pharmacists in England and Wales.

Essential services must be provided by all community pharmacies and are not open to local negotiation. The list of essential services includes:

- dispensing of medicines
- repeat dispensing
- disposal of unwanted medicines
- public health
- signposting
- self-care
- clinical governance.

Advanced services require both the pharmacist and the pharmacy premises to be accredited and include a medicines use review (MUR) and prescription intervention (PI) service. Practical issues surrounding the provision of an MUR service will be discussed in Chapter 5.

Enhanced services are commissioned locally by primary care trusts (PCTs). A service specification (for England) or a national enhanced service template (Wales) and a fee for providing the service will be agreed nationally. In 2005–2006, the enhanced services most frequently provided were:[3]

- stop-smoking support service
- supervised administration of medicines
- minor ailments schemes
- supply of medicines via patient group directions.

The practicalities of offering enhanced services will be discussed in Chapter 6.

Implications for social care

It is expected that the new contractual arrangements will contribute a number of benefits to the social care service. Examples of areas of the contract that may impact on social care include:

- MUR service that aims to improve the way that people use their medicines may help to reduce the number of hospital admissions as a result of inappropriate use of medicines
- repeat-dispensing service will provide a more convenient service for both patients and carers, and reduce the need to visit the general practitioner (GP) every time a supply of medication is needed
- the support offered through the essential service of self-care through the management of minor ailments and conditions will offer more choice and access to those who wish to care for themselves or their families.
- under the Disability Discrimination Act 1995 (DDA), pharmacists will offer additional support for patients who require help in taking their medicines due to a disability, for example by providing reminder charts, large-print labels or other compliance aids

■ signposting by pharmacists to other health and social care providers may offer a more co-ordinated approach to the referral of patients to the appropriate service provider

■ there will be a formal arrangement for the disposal of unwanted medicines and this will ensure that medicines are less likely to accumulate in the home and community

■ locally commissioned enhanced services will encourage the development of new and innovative pharmacy services and it may be that there is the possibility of increased collaborative working between pharmacy services and social services.

Essential services

Essential service 1: dispensing of medicines

There are two main aims of the essential dispensing service:

■ to ensure that medicines are dispensed safely. This will involve the appropriate, legal, clinical and accuracy checks when a prescription is presented

■ to ensure the patient knows how to use the dispensed item. This will involve the provision of appropriate advice including broader information about potential side-effects and interactions.

The service specification for this essential service states that the pharmacy must maintain a record of all medicines and appliances supplied, which can be used to assist patient care.[4] In addition the pharmacy should maintain a record of any advice given, and interventions and referrals made, where the pharmacist judges it to be clinically appropriate.

One of the key issues in the provision of a reliable and consistent dispensing service is the use of well-written standard operating procedures (SOPs). The use of SOPs is discussed later in this chapter.

Essential service 2: repeat dispensing

Repeatable prescriptions have been limited by NHS regulations and reimbursement processes. In April 2004 legislation came into force to enable prescribing doctors, independent nurse prescribers and all supplementary prescribers to issue repeatable prescriptions. This legislation allows pharmacists to dispense and be reimbursed for repeatable prescriptions under the NHS. The aims of this essential service are to:

■ increase patient choice and convenience

■ minimise wastage by reducing the amount of dispensed unwanted medicine

- reduce the workload of general medical practice
- make greater use of pharmacists' skills.

The Centre for Pharmacy Postgraduate Education (CPPE) distance learning pack *Repeat Dispensing from Pathfinder to Practice* was circulated to all pharmacists in England and outlines the stages of the repeat-dispensing process.[5] The slightly different repeat-dispensing arrangements in Wales are covered in the WCPPE package.[6]

The nine stages involved in offering a repeat-dispensing service can be summarised as follows:

1 Selecting suitable patients

Repeat dispensing is a partnership between the patient, prescriber and pharmacist; not all patients will benefit from this service. In selecting suitable patients for repeat dispensing, the criteria used are:

- patients with long-term conditions
- patients with conditions that are likely to remain stable during the repeat-dispensing period.

In practice different GP surgeries have different approaches to selecting patients. For example some surgeries may target all patients on a particular drug such as levothyroxine. Another approach is to select patients who have recently had a medication review and are stable on a number of medicines. The pharmacist needs to be aware of the selection criteria that are being used locally so that they can contribute to the selection process and ensure that patients are aware of the availability of this service.

2 Gaining patient consent

Participation in a repeat-dispensing service is voluntary and some patients may prefer to remain with their existing dispensing arrangements. As there will be exchange of information about the patient's medication or treatment between the GP and the pharmacist, the patient needs to give fully informed consent before participating in this service. The patient must be fully informed of the process and provided with written material of how the system operates so that they can make an informed decision. Medical practice reception staff are generally responsible for this process. The pharmacist needs to be aware of the arrangements that exist for approaching patients to consider this service at local medical practices. Agreement by the patient is then recorded on an agreement form and a copy retained on the patient's file in the surgery.

3 Managing receipt of a repeatable prescription and associated batch issues

The repeat-dispensing system consists of a repeatable prescription which is signed by the prescriber and also a number of batch prescriptions which are not signed. The repeatable prescription forms the legal prescription for the repeat supply of the medication. The unsigned batch prescriptions act as invoice for the pharmacist to receive payment for making each supply of medication. When the repeat prescription is first presented the pharmacist should explain the process so that the patient is fully aware of the practical details involved.

A clinical and legal check is made of the repeatable prescription and the first batch prescription is dispensed. The prescriber needs to specify the number of instalments allowed on the prescription. In some cases the prescriber may specify the instalment interval, and in many cases this will be monthly. However the instalment interval can be flexible and does not need to be stated. It is expected that the pharmacist will use professional judgement to dispense instalments at an appropriate time. The repeatable prescription will need to be retained by the pharmacy for the duration of the dispensing period.

If a patient wishes to change pharmacy then they will need to be referred back to the prescriber. All medicines can be supplied under the repeat-dispensing arrangements with the exception of Schedules 2 and 3 controlled drugs. A repeatable prescription must be dispensed for the first time within 6 months of being written and is valid for a period of 12 months from this date unless an earlier expiry is specified by the prescriber.

4 Referral of any medicine-management issues

During the repeat-dispensing period it is part of the regulations that pharmacists and prescribers will need to contact each other in certain circumstances. For example there may be issues reported by the pharmacist such as compliance problems, adverse reactions or medicines-management issues. The GP will need to inform the pharmacist of any changes to medication or if changes are required to prescribed items. The pharmacist will need to be fully informed of local arrangements for this referral process and ensure measures are in place to maintain a closed loop communication system.

5 Endorsement of the prescription

The repeatable prescription is stamped in the usual way with the name and address of the pharmacy. The batch issues are endorsed with quantities and items dispensed as specified by the *Drug Tariff*. A clear audit trail of dispensed items needs to be in place and this will involve keeping a record that can be clearly linked to the repeatable prescription. Many pharmacies attach a record card to the repeatable prescription that records the dates and quantities supplied of each item.

6 Re-imbursement of batch issues supplied

Batch issue forms are submitted with other prescriptions for re-imbursement to the NHS Business Services Authority, Prescription Pricing Division (PPD). Any batch issues that have not been dispensed within the repeat-dispensing period should be destroyed and a record made of the destruction.

7 Storage of repeatable prescriptions and batch issues if requested by the patient

Many pharmacies find the management of the repeat-dispensing process easier if a designated storage area is used for the repeatable prescriptions. In practice this may mean using a lockable filing cabinet and assigning a member of the dispensing team to manage the process. Repeat items should be prepared in advance, to avoid the patient having to wait for their medication. The repeatable prescription must be retained at the pharmacy. The batch issues may be retained by the patient to bring in when they require their repeat medication. In most cases the patient prefers to leave all the prescription forms at the pharmacy.

8 Making the final instalment

When the patient collects their last instalment they need to be reminded to make an appointment so that the prescriber may review their condition, and if appropriate issue another repeatable prescription and set of batch issues. Some pharmacists use a standard written reminder form to facilitate this process.

9 Final submission of the repeatable prescription to the PPD

The repeatable prescription is finally submitted to the PPD separately from the batch issues in the month after it has expired. The repeatable prescription would be submitted to the PPD earlier if there have been medication changes that make the form no longer valid.

A repeat-dispensing SOP should be developed for each pharmacy taking into account arrangements with local surgeries. After testing and modification the SOP should be made widely available to all temporary staff to ensure the smooth running of this essential service.

The service specification for the repeat-dispensing service specifies the following:[7]

- pharmacy contractors are required to undertake appropriate training to ensure they are competent to deliver this service
- specific arrangements must be in place to ensure that there is direct communication to locum pharmacists to ensure that they are aware of the practical local procedures in place
- pharmacy staff will be required to communicate with patients about how the repeat-dispensing system operates and the importance of ordering only prescription items that are required
- the pharmacy will store the patient's documentation securely
- the pharmacist is expected to use their professional judgement to decide if it is appropriate for the item to be dispensed
- it is the responsibility of the pharmacist prior to supplying the repeat medication to ensure that the patient is using the medicine appropriately and there are no side-effects that would require a review of the treatment. The pharmacist should also check if there have been any other changes that would suggest that a medication review by the prescriber would be beneficial
- each batch issue prescription should be endorsed appropriately and forwarded to the PPD as specified in the *Drug Tariff*
- the pharmacist may refuse to dispense the batch issue if they are concerned about safety, for example if there has been a change in the patient's medical condition or medication
- there must be a clear audit trail so that pharmacy staff can easily determine the dates and quantities of medicines supplied at each dispensing. Any clinically significant interventions should be recorded and maintained in the patient's record
- the prescriber should be informed by the pharmacist of any issues of clinical significance that relate to the repeatable prescription.

Essential service 3: disposal of unwanted medicines

The disposal of unwanted medicines is an essential service that aims to provide the public with an easy and safe method of disposing of unwanted medicines. The service should reduce the risk to the public in the following ways:

- reduce the quantity of stored unwanted medicine in people's homes and reduce the risk of accidental poisonings
- reduce the risk of exposure to medicines that have been disposed of by non-secure methods
- reduced environmental damage caused by inappropriate disposal methods for unwanted medicines.

Community pharmacists should be aware of the following issues that surround this essential service:

- PCT responsibility
- pharmacy as a collection point
- storage of waste
- segregation of waste
- waste pharmacy medicines
- waste-management legislation
- clinical waste.

PCT responsibility

A pharmacy does not have to start providing the service until the PCT has made suitable arrangements for collecting unwanted medicines from the pharmacy. This will involve the use of a specialist waste contractor that will regularly collect waste from the pharmacy. The PCT will need to register as a broker for the collection and disposal of medicines with the local environment agency.

Pharmacy as a collection point

As a collection point for waste, the pharmacy can collect unwanted medicines from the public. The public is defined as individuals and residential care homes. The provision for using the pharmacy as a waste-collection point does not include nursing homes or waste from a general medical practice as this waste is defined as industrial clinical waste.

Storage of waste

The waste-disposal contractor will provide the pharmacy with approved containers and all waste must be stored in these containers.

Segregation of waste

Waste should be segregated into four types:

- solid dosage-form medicines and ampoules
- liquids – stored in a special liquid waste container
- aerosols
- Schedules 2 and 3 controlled drugs (CDs) should be denatured before disposing as the waste contractor is not authorised to possess a CD. It is important that waste CDs are stored in a CD cabinet until the items are denatured and therefore are no longer classified as a CD. At present the Environment Agency regard the denaturing of CDs as a low-risk activity

and deem it is not necessary to have a waste-management licence to carry out this procedure.[8]

Waste pharmacy medicines

The Special Waste Regulations 1996 specify that different categories of waste should not be mixed. Different categories of medicine for the purpose of waste disposal can be defined by the following list:

- waste medicine items returned by the public
- waste medicines from a pharmacy such as dispensing stock that is out of date
- waste prescription only medicines from a pharmacy are classified as special waste and cannot be mixed with pharmacy (P) or general sales list (GSL) medicines.

If P or GSL medicines have hazardous properties, for example if they are flammable, oxidising, irritant, harmful, toxic or corrosive, they are regarded as special waste.

It is a requirement that waste medicines that have originated from a pharmacy will not be mixed with waste items handed in by the public for disposal.

Waste-management legislation

The community pharmacist needs to be aware of the relevant waste-management legislation and ensure the following measures are in place:

- the pharmacy premises are registered with the local office of the Environment Agency as exempt from the Waste Management Licensing (WML) Regulations 1994 as they are storing waste medicines returned from the public
- if the pharmacy employs a driver to collect waste medicines from patients' homes, the driver will need to be registered as a waste carrier with the local office of the Environment Agency. This would include the driver bringing unwanted medicines from a residential home
- the secure storage of waste medicines should not exceed $5m^3$ at any one time and the storage should be for no longer than 6 months at a time.
- the pharmacy will need to retain descriptions and transfer notes of waste collected for at least 2 years. Any special waste-management consignment notes will have to be retained on a register for at least 3 years
- the pharmacy contractor will need to make staff aware of the risks associated with handling waste medicines. Pharmacy staff will need appropriate protective equipment and clothing and materials to deal with any spillages. It would be expected that there are gloves, overalls and suitable materials available to deal with spillages near to the area where the waste medicines are stored.

Clinical waste

Diagnostic testing in the pharmacy can generate a certain amount of clinical waste such as used sharps and swabs for finger prick blood tests. Needle-exchange schemes also involve the storage and disposal of contaminated sharps. This type of clinical waste is defined as a separate category to medicines waste and can be collected from the pharmacy by a licensed waste disposal contractor. A full waste-management licence is not required for this activity.

Essential service 4: promotion of healthy lifestyles

Public health has always been a part of the community pharmacist's agenda and there is an increasing emphasis on this role. Pharmacists will play a key role in the 'health-promoting NHS' as outlined in the Government's white paper *Choosing Health: making healthy choices easier.*[9] This role is expanded further in the document: *Choosing Health through Pharmacy. A programme for pharmaceutical public health 2005–2015.*[10] An overview of some of the areas of pharmacist involvement is summarised in Figure 4.2.

Promoting healthy lifestyles consists of two separate areas:

- prescription-linked intervention
- involvement in public health campaigns.

Prescription-linked intervention involves offering opportunistic advice on public health topics to patients that present a prescription. Offering public health advice has always been part of the role of a community pharmacist, and the new contract aims to formalise pharmacist input in this area. Promotion of healthy lifestyles will include offering advice when patients from any of the following groups present a prescription:

- patients with diabetes
- people at risk of coronary heart disease such as smokers, those with high blood pressure and those who are overweight.

It is expected that pharmacists will have a structured discussion about relevant health issues such as stopping smoking, recommended alcohol intake, nutrition advice and the importance of increased physical activity. The verbal advice should be backed up by written information such as leaflets if necessary, and the advice given will be recorded on the patient's pharmacy record. The record will allow the pharmacist to follow the progress of individual patients, follow up the consultation with further advice, and facilitate audit of this service.

Systems and procedures need to be in place to ensure that appropriate advice is given to patients. This may include the use of appropriate

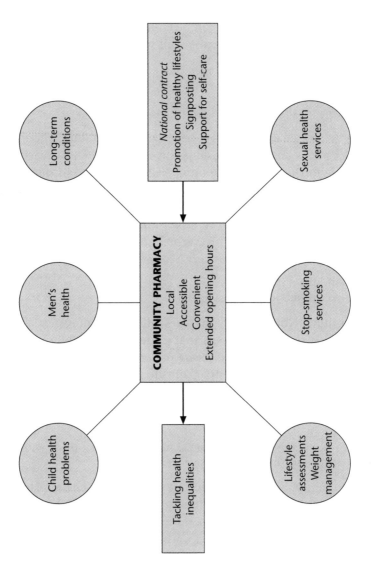

Figure 4.2 Pharmacist involvement in the promotion of healthy lifestyles.

reminder prompts on the patient medication record (PMR) system such as a prompt to ask open questions regarding lifestyle, when new prescriptions are presented for antihypertensive drugs.

The involvement in public health campaigns will be decided by the individual PCT. Public health campaigns aim to engage the pharmacist in promoting key healthy lifestyle messages, especially to hard-to-reach sectors of the population. It is envisaged that the pharmacist will be involved in up to six public health campaigns each year. During the campaign pharmacy staff will be proactive in providing public health information to both patients and general visitors to the pharmacy. A record of the number of people who receive advice related to the campaign should be recorded.

The essential service of promoting healthy lifestyles is linked to two other essential services: signposting and supporting self care.

Essential service 5: signposting

The community pharmacist has always provided the public with information about other agencies that can provide additional support, advice or treatment. The essential service of signposting patients in this way is now formalised in the national contract. The aims of this service are to:

- inform or advise people who require assistance from health and/or social care providers
- enable people to access further care and support appropriate to their needs
- minimise inappropriate use of health and social care services.

It is the responsibility of the PCT to provide the pharmacy with referral contact details of appropriate health and social care providers such as local patient groups. To comply with this service it is expected that pharmacy staff will inform or advise people visiting the pharmacy of where to find extra support to meet their health and social needs. In some cases a written referral note may be provided to the patient if this is deemed to be necessary. If the pharmacist makes a judgement that the advice given to the patient is of clinical significance and the patient is known to the pharmacy staff, then a record of the signposting advice may be made on the patient's pharmacy record.

Essential service 6: support for self-care

In common with signposting and promoting healthy lifestyles, the support of people requesting advice on self-care is a well-established role for the community pharmacist. The aims and intended outcomes of this essential service as described in the service specification are to provide people and their carers with enhanced choice and access to support for self-care.[11] This involves providing people and their carers with:

- appropriate advice to help them manage self-limiting or long-term conditions, including advice on the selection and use of non-prescription medicines
- health-promotion advice in line with advice provided in other essential services
- information and advice about treatment options, including non-pharmacological options to enable improved self-management of conditions.

This service will involve pharmacy staff in providing management advice and information on both minor illness and long-term conditions. The advice to people and their carers will include information on non-prescription medicines and opportunistic healthy lifestyle interventions. Self-care referrals are received by community pharmacists from NHS Direct and other healthcare professionals. In common with the signposting essential service, community pharmacists will direct patients to other health and social care providers. A record on the patient's pharmacy record will be made if the patient is known to the pharmacy staff and the pharmacist deems the advice to be of clinical significance. The record should include any advice given, products purchased or details of any referrals made.

Essential service 7: clinical governance requirements

The community pharmacy contract is based on quality; therefore compliance with clinical governance requirements is an essential service. This essential service specifies that all community pharmacies have an identifiable clinical governance lead and apply clinical governance principles to the delivery of all services. This lead person does not necessarily have to be a pharmacist.

There are three principles of clinical governance in relation to the community pharmacy contract:

- clinical governance (continuous quality improvement) should be embedded into all professional services
- clinical governance is driven by a genuine desire to improve the service delivered to patients
- the development of clinical governance should be supported and encouraged by primary care organisations.

The Healthcare Commission promotes quality in healthcare through providing an independent assessment of the standards of services provided by the NHS, private healthcare and voluntary organisations. There are seven components of clinical governance as used by the Healthcare Commission to assess how well an organisation meets clinical governance requirements. All of these requirements are embedded into the activities of the pharmacy that impact on patient care. Each component will be considered separately, but it should be recognised that there is a significant overlap between these areas. The seven areas are summarised in Figure 4.3.

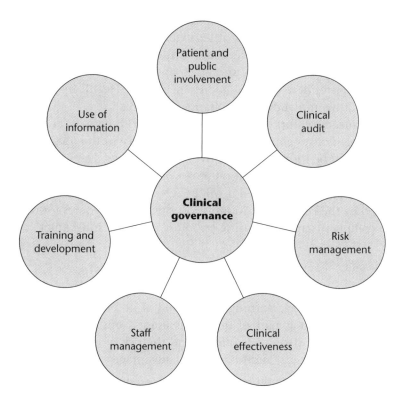

Figure 4.3 Overview of the clinical governance requirements for the community pharmacy contract.

Patient and public involvement

The first requirement of the clinical governance section of the contract is that pharmacies should have a practice leaflet that will inform patients of the NHS services offered by the pharmacy. Community pharmacy contractors will also have to annually administer a patient satisfaction survey. The survey is based on a national template and asks for feedback from patients on the promptness of supply, quality of service and quality of facilities. The minimum number of returned surveys required is dependent on the average monthly prescription volume. It is expected that the pharmacist will review the surveys and make improvements where necessary. Patient and public involvement with community pharmacy will also include visits from local patient and public involvement forums, which are made up of volunteers and exist in every PCT in England. The role of patient and public involvement forums is to independently monitor service providers. The NHS trust has a legal obligation to respond to the issues raised by this monitoring activity. The contractor is also expected to work with other external organisations such as the Healthcare Commission and local authorities. Similar arrangements exist in Wales where the pharmacy should co-operate with local health boards and other appropriate external bodies such as the Health Inspectorate in the monitoring and auditing of pharmacy services.

As a means of improving communication with patients and the public, a complaints system should already be in place in the pharmacy. This system should be formalised and involves two stages. The first stage is to bring a complaint to the attention of the practitioner or the organisation. If the complaint is unresolved it will be referred to the second stage to be managed by the Healthcare Commission. Specific procedures for responding to complaints and dispensing errors are discussed in Chapter 7.

Clinical audit

A simple definition of audit is 'improving the care of patients by looking at what you are doing, learning from it and, if necessary, changing practice'. Clinical audit is part of quality assurance, ensuring that the best possible service to patients is offered and the risk of errors minimised.[12] Involvement in clinical audit has several advantages:

- it demonstrates a willingness to maintain good professional standards
- it improves the quality of working life
- it enhances the efficient use of resources
- it helps to support change by producing objective information about the quality of care.

The objective of an audit needs to be clearly stated, for example:

> To ensure that all members of the pharmacy team provide appropriate and up-to-date information when they receive requests for weight-management advice.

Contractors are expected to participate in two clinical audits each year to comply with this component of clinical governance. One audit is practice based and the other audit involves a multidisciplinary approach which is determined by the PCT. Both audits must have a clear outcome and be used to contribute to the development of patient care. Both clinical audits should be able to be completed within 5 days of pharmacist time, and it is expected that the PCT will give the pharmacist adequate notice of any meetings involved in the multidisciplinary audit so that they can make arrangements to leave the pharmacy premises.

Risk management

The management of risk covers a diverse range of activities in the pharmacy and the service specification covers the following areas:

- stock-sourcing and handling procedures
- equipment maintenance
- patient safety incident log for reporting to the National Patient Safety Agency (NPSA)
- analysis and monitoring of critical incidents
- root cause analysis
- standard operating procedures for many of the pharmacy's functions
- waste-disposal systems for clinical and confidential waste
- compliance with health and safety legislation and child-protection procedures.

Clinical effectiveness

Clinical effectiveness is a general term used to describe a range of activities that help the healthcare professional to measure, monitor and improve the quality of patient care that they provide. This is not the same as clinical governance but forms part of clinical governance. For the community pharmacist to practise in a clinically effective way, they must ensure that they work within best current practice and evidence-based guidelines for all patient and customer interactions. This will involve working within policies that are intended to manage risk and reduce harm to patients.

To ensure that appropriate self-care advice is given there should be systems in place such as protocols, SOPs and algorithms. Pharmacies should also contribute to the clinical effectiveness of prescribing through the management of repeatable prescriptions and the MUR service. To demonstrate clinical effectiveness, the pharmacist will need to maintain accurate records and undertake clinical audit to demonstrate improvement in their practice.

Staff management

It is a requirement that all contractors ensure that all pharmacy staff and locum pharmacists are provided with induction training that covers issues such as confidentiality, health and safety and security. All staff members are provided with training that is appropriate to their role and there is support for their ongoing development needs. When employing new staff who are providing NHS services, references should be taken up and all qualifications checked. A list of employed pharmacists and locums will be held by the PCT.

Training and development

Pharmacists will have to be able to demonstrate a commitment to continuing professional development (CPD) using a CPD record in line with the Royal Pharmaceutical Society of Great Britain (RPSGB) requirements. There is a requirement for pharmacists to become accredited before providing advanced or enhanced services.

Use of information

It is expected that pharmacy staff will be able to access up to date reference sources such as the *British National Formulary* (BNF) and *Drug Tariff* and have appropriate IT links to electronic reference sources. Confidentiality policies need to be in place to protect patient data and confidentiality. Full records of any interventions and advice given should be made where this will improve patient care. The pharmacy will also need to provide the PCT and NHS Direct with updated information on their opening hours.

Standard operating procedures (SOPs)

From January 2005 the RPSGB required all pharmacies to have written SOPs covering the dispensing process. This requirement applies to both hospital and community sectors and covers all of the activities which occur from the time that prescriptions are received in the pharmacy or by a pharmacist until medicines or other prescribed items have been collected or transferred to the patient.[13]

A SOP is a written document that specifies what should be done, when, where and by whom. The RPSGB consultation document on SOPs in a community pharmacy stated that SOPs have the following benefits:[14]

- help to assure the quality of the service
- help to ensure that good practice is achieved consistently
- enable pharmacists to delegate more readily and may possibly free the pharmacist's time for other activities

- help to avoid confusion over who does what and clarify roles within the pharmacy
- provide advice and guidance to locums and part-time staff
- provide useful training tools for new members of staff
- provide a contribution to the audit process.

The main driver behind the introduction of SOPs is the compliance with clinical governance requirements to put in place strategies for risk management and risk minimisation. Pharmacists are accountable for the dispensing process but the development of SOPs will allow pharmacists to examine current dispensing practice and benchmark good practice in this area.

There are three general principles that apply to all SOPs:

- the SOP must be pharmacy specific. There is wide recognition that pharmacies vary considerably in their working environment and the SOP will be specific to a pharmacy
- the SOP will depend on the competence of the staff working in a specific pharmacy. For example there may be more stages and more explanation in the SOP where there are lower numbers of competent staff
- the SOP will be applicable at all times in a specific pharmacy. The SOP should not be dependent on the presence of the pharmacist under whose authority the procedure was prepared.

Anatomy of an SOP

Each SOP has two main parts:

The first part is an outline or summary that includes:

- *the aim or purpose* of the overall SOP
- *objectives* – what is the procedure trying to achieve?
- *scope* – what areas of work are to be covered by the procedure?
- *risks* – are there any risks associated with the task?
- *review date* – to ensure that the procedure continues to be useful and up to date

The second or main part of the document includes:

- *stages of the process* – describe how the task is to be carried out step by step
- *responsibility* – who is responsible for carrying out each stage of the process: (1) under normal operating conditions; (2) in different circumstances, for example when staff are on holiday or there is a computer failure
- *other useful information* – is there any other information that could usefully be included in the procedure? Does the SOP incorporate mechanisms for audit?

A specific example of an SOP for waste disposal is provided in Figure 4.4.

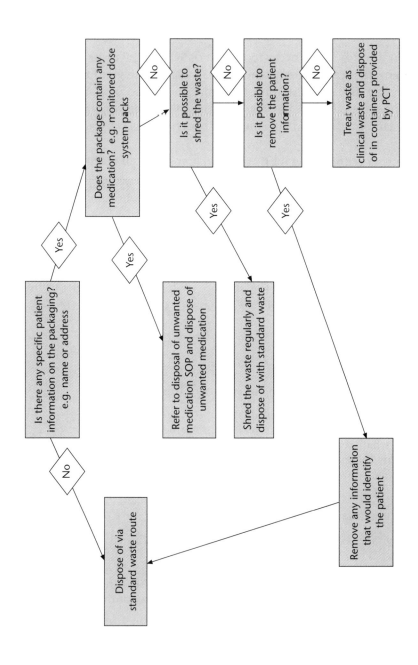

Figure 4.4 Standard operating procedure (SOP) in a flow chart format for the *confidential* waste disposal of medicines other than controlled drugs.

For the purposes of writing an SOP the RPSGB has divided the dispensing process into six main steps:

- taking in prescriptions
- pharmaceutical assessment
- interventions and problem solving
- assembly and labelling
- accuracy checking
- transfer to the patient.

As a minimum, all of these six areas should be covered by SOPs. Individual pharmacies will then go on to develop SOPs for areas that are specific to their practice. Examples that may be relevant for an individual pharmacy include:

- dispensing methadone or other items to drug users
- providing services to nursing or residential care homes
- prescription collection and delivery services
- telephone requests for prescriptions
- the use of child-resistant containers (CRCs)
- recording interventions
- queries from other healthcare professionals
- supply of specials
- dealing with 'owings', including the procedure to be followed at the time of the second dispensing.

Top tips for producing SOPs[15]

- Take into account practical variables such as sickness, holidays, volume of work and the resources available.
- Avoid long wordy instructions. Keep the stages small and simple to follow.
- Use diagrams and flow charts where possible.
- Cross reference to other information such as 'in house' training manuals or documents or computer manuals.
- Experiment with different layouts such as using algorithms or the use of bulleted points
- Involve different members of staff in the writing process. The accountability for the SOP is with the pharmacist but it is useful to have input into the writing process.
- Decide if responsible staff will be named on the SOP or whether job titles will be used, for example 'dispenser' or 'counter assistant'
- Make sure the SOP matches the layout and workflow of the pharmacy. For example an unusual dispensary layout may mean that the SOP for assembling and labelling needs to be very specific for the SOP to work. A specific SOP also informs locum staff of the differences in procedures in an individual pharmacy.

continued overleaf

■ Keep all SOPs in a designated folder and also give out copies to members of staff who are involved in the dispensing process. Make sure that locum staff can access the information easily.

■ Allow all members of staff to become involved once the SOP has been drafted, and invite comments. Trial the SOP for a few months and modify the procedure according to input from the pharmacy team. The review date will be stated on the SOP document and should be at least annually. Change the SOP before the review date if there is a dispensing error related to the SOP or there is a change in company procedure or legislation changes.

Pharmacists working for a large organisation will be supplied with SOP templates from their central office that require local adaptation. The template is then adapted by each pharmacy to specify how each task is done, which member of staff is responsible and what level of training the person performing the task must have. There is usually the facility for local stores to opt out of this system and produce their own SOP, which will then require approval by the superintendent pharmacist or their representative.

If a pharmacist works for an independent pharmacy they are starting with a clean sheet of paper. The advantage in this is that the pharmacist can take individual circumstances of their pharmacy into account from the outset.

There are various sources of support for pharmacists writing SOPs:

■ the RPSGB website provides guidance on writing SOPs for the six dispensing steps[16]

■ the Centre for Pharmacy Postgraduate Education (CPPE) has a multimedia distance learning package called SWEEP. This package is aimed at helping pharmacists write a variety of SOPs within the pharmacy and not confined to the area of dispensing

■ National Pharmacy Association (NPA) members can access a training package developed in conjunction with GlaxoSmithKline's Plus programme.

Monitoring of the contract

Compliance of pharmacy contractors with the national contract in England is monitored by the PCT. It is suggested that the PCT involve the local pharmaceutical committee (LPC) to discuss the format of the monitoring process. In most cases the monitoring visit by the PCT is an annual visit to the pharmacy premises.

The NHS Primary Care Contracting (PCC) monitoring toolkit[17] is generally used as the basis for monitoring the contract. This consists of a nationally designed and agreed format of indicators and quality markers that a pharmacy can be measured against.

To assist the contractor in preparing for the contract, reference can be made to the PSNC *New Contract Workbook*.[18] This document contains full details of the contract and assists the contractor to collate important information that may be required during the monitoring visit. The PCC monitoring toolkit contains a self-assessment tool that enables the contractor to assess compliance with different parts of the contract. A series of statements under the different essential services are self-assessed by the contractor as: always doing (green), mostly doing (amber) and rarely doing (red). Examples of self-assessment monitoring statements include:

- 'All prescriptions have legal, clinical and accuracy checks'
- 'Appropriate protective equipment and spillage kits are available for staff to use'.

The monitoring visit should not impact on the running of the pharmacy or disrupt the concentration of the pharmacy staff. It is important that the visit is prepared for and all the necessary documentation is to hand. A formative self-assessment by the contractor may reduce the amount of time spent on the actual visit and also the breadth of the visit. After the visit, the pharmacy contractor should be given a minimum of 3 months' written notice to rectify any areas of non-compliance, before any action is taken. Guidelines on non-compliance with the contract are provided in a Department of Health briefing paper.[19]

Support for people with disabilities

The new contract initially proposed an essential service entitled 'Support for people with disabilities'. This service was not included in the new contractual framework. However, under the Disability Discrimination Act 1995 (DDA),[20] pharmacists providing services in the UK have a legal obligation to make reasonable adjustments to their services and provide auxiliary aids where appropriate for people with disabilities.

Before the DDA there was a register of disabled persons that was maintained under Section 6 of the Disabled Persons (Employment) Act 1944. A person on the register for a period of 3 years was deemed to be a disabled person within the meaning of this Act. There is now no register on which a person with a disability is recorded. For example before the

DDA a person may have been registered disabled for reasons such as difficulty in walking, becoming easily tired, or conditions such as emphysema. All of these conditions could satisfy the former definition of a disabled person but the person would not necessarily have difficulties with their medicines.

Under the DDA a person is considered disabled if he, or she, has a mental, sensory or physical impairment that would have a substantial and long-term adverse effect on his or her ability to carry out normal day-to-day activities.[21]

The DDA will apply if at least one of the following is affected by the impairment:

- mobility
- manual dexterity
- physical co-ordination
- continence
- ability to lift, carry or otherwise move everyday objects
- speech hearing or eyesight
- memory or ability to concentrate, learn or understand
- perception of the risk of physical danger.

The DDA has been amended to cover conditions such as cancer, HIV and multiple sclerosis that cause an intermittent disability or progressive disability. The amendment has also removed the criteria for a mental impairment to be clinically recognised.

The following requirements apply to pharmacy services under the DDA:[22]

- disabled people should not be treated less favourably than other people for any reason related to their disability
- reasonable adjustments for disabled people include providing extra help or changing the way that services are provided
- reasonable adjustments to the physical features of pharmacy premises to overcome barriers to access should be made.

A contribution for the adjustments made by pharmacies for patients eligible under the DDA is made within the practice payment received by the pharmacy and detailed in the *Drug Tariff*.[23] Provision for the payment of auxiliary aids for patients not eligible under the DDA will not be covered. In some cases patients not covered by the DDA will be covered by negotiated arrangements with the PCT or social services.

There are two stages for a community pharmacist when considering their service provision to people with disabilities:

1 to assess the patient to confirm that they are covered by the DDA
2 to decide what reasonable adjustments are needed in order to comply with the DDA.

An example of different patients with disabilities and how they may affect their access to pharmacy services is provided in Table 4.1.

Table 4.1 Examples of patients with disabilities and how they may affect their access to pharmacy services

Patient	Is the person disabled within the meaning of the Act?	Are they are able to access pharmacy services (medicines)?
Person with severe arthritis	Yes	A child-resistant container would be unreasonably difficult or impossible for this patient
Person who cannot walk unaided	Yes	No particular constraints on the use of medicines
Person with short-term memory loss that has a substantial impact on day-to-day living	Yes	Loose medicines in a bottle may be a problem. The supply of a calendar pack or monitored dosage system may improve compliance

The assessment of the patient could involve an informal discussion, or a more formal approach can be adopted by using assessment forms. One of the assessment tools for pharmacy contractors has been commissioned by the Department of Health on the NHS Primary Care Contracting website.[24] In some cases the use of a variety of other assessment methods may be more appropriate. The assessment must be carried out in a suitable environment that offers privacy and confidentiality. The following issues should be considered when carrying out a patient assessment:

- assessments should ignore corrective interventions that have been made to support a disability. The exception to this is visual impairment which should only be assessed when the patient is using spectacles or contact lenses. If large-print labels are being considered it may be appropriate to refer the patient to an optometrist for an updated eye check
- the disease may have progressed, even though symptoms have improved, and the patient may need reassessment
- communication pathways with other health and social care professionals should be developed. In some cases the pharmacist will be unable to support the patient appropriately and will need to be able to signpost the patient to a health and social care assessment or a local support group.

The next stage is to decide what reasonable adjustments are required by the patient, in order to access the services being offered. Potentially a difficult situation can arise if the patient demands or believes that they need a particular adjustment to the service and the patient assessment demonstrates that this is not necessary.

Examples of reasonable adjustments to dispensing services include:

- removing tablets from packaging if the patient is unable to remove tablets from blister packs
- providing wing caps for patients who are unable to open ordinary screw caps
- provision of pen and paper to facilitate communication if the patient is unable to speak clearly
- supplying smaller lighter-weight plastic liquid medicine bottles for patients who have difficulty pouring from a large heavy glass bottle.

There are numerous examples of reasonable adjustments, and it is important that the pharmacist works in partnership with the patient to negotiate a reasonable approach to supplying their medicines. For example it may be considered unreasonable for the pharmacist to install an expensive hearing loop or purchase a Braille typewriter to produce Braille labels for the visually impaired. These are examples of situations where the PCT may have to commission a locally enhanced service to cater for the needs of patients who require these costly adjustments.

Community pharmacy contract for Scotland

The Scottish contract for community pharmacists differs from the contract in England and Wales. The contract is based on four core services: an acute medication service (AMS), a minor ailment service (MAS), a chronic medication service (CMS) and a public health service (PHS).[25] Unlike the contract for England and Wales the contract is effectively a single tier that consists of four services that all community pharmacists in Scotland must provide. Any additional services such as harm-reduction services, care home services, out-of-hours services and waste collection are to be agreed locally but will be based on national specifications. The Scottish contract, in common with England and Wales, also underlines making better use of pharmacists' skills and the development of pharmacy services. The Scottish Executive's 10-year plan for NHS Scotland emphasises the value of community pharmacists based in local communities and the importance of public health and preventative healthcare.[26] The main focus of the contract is on the provision of pharmaceutical care.

In summary, the four core services include:

- *acute medication service* (AMS) which is essentially the regular dispensing service
- *minor ailment service* (MAS) that offers patients who are exempt from prescription charges the provision of having minor ailments treated free of charge in the pharmacy. This will involve the patient in registering with a pharmacy via an electronic central patient registration system
- *chronic medication service* (CMS) that involves a pharmacist in the management of a patient's long-term medication for up to 12 months. This will include the provision of medicines and the associated monitoring and reviewing of medicines. In some cases there will be a shared care agreement between the patient the GP and the community pharmacist. Payment for the CMS will be on a capitation basis
- *public health service* (PHS) which includes the provision of information on public health issues and the participation in national and local public health campaigns. There is an emphasis on using the community pharmacy network as healthy living walk-in centres to communicate healthy lifestyle messages to local communities.

The Scottish contract was introduced in April 2006 and a phased implementation process is planned as supporting information management and technology becomes available.

Implications for practice

Activity 1

- Visit the audit section of the RPSGB website: www.rpsgb.org.uk/registrationandsupport/audit/index.html
- Examine the audit templates and consider designing a new audit that is particularly relevant to your current practice.

Activity 2

Carry out a review of a minimum of three different SOPs that are commonly used in your practice. Ask your pharmacy team for their comments on each SOP under the following headings:

- compliance with SOP
- ease of use
- suggested improvements (if any).

- Are there any common themes that emerge from this assessment?
- Modify the SOPs to take into account any suggested improvements.

Multiple choice questions

Directions for question 1: each of the questions or incomplete statements in this section is followed by five suggested answers. Select the best answer in each case.

Q1 Which of the following services requires accreditation of the pharmacist and premises?

A Disposal of unwanted medicines
B Promoting healthy lifestyles
C Medicines use review
D Repeat dispensing
E Signposting

Directions for questions 2 and 3: for each numbered question select the one lettered option above it which is most closely related to it. Within each group of questions each lettered option may be used once, more than once, or not at all.

A Prescription intervention service
B Minor-ailments service
C Repeat dispensing
D Clinical governance
E Support for self-care

Select from A to E which one of the above fits the following statements

Q2 An advanced service
Q3 An enhanced service

Directions for questions 4 to 8: each of the questions or incomplete statements in this section is followed by three responses. For each question ONE or MORE of the responses is (are) correct. Decide which of the responses is (are) correct. Then choose:

A if 1, 2 and 3 are correct
B if 1 and 2 only are correct
C if 2 and 3 only are correct
D if 1 only is correct
E if 3 only is correct

Directions summarised:
A: 1, 2, 3   B: 1, 2 only   C: 2, 3 only   D: 1 only   E: 3 only

Q4 Which of the following organisations were involved in negotiation for the contractual framework for community pharmacy?

1 Department of Health

2   NHS Confederation
3   PSNC

Q5 Which of the following statements about essential services in the contract for England and Wales is (are) correct?

1   They are provided by all pharmacies.
2   The services are not open to local negotiation.
3   There must be the provision of a MUR service.

Q6 Which of the following statements about the dispensing service is (are) correct?

1   All prescriptions should have a legal, clinical and accuracy check.
2   The pharmacy must make a record of all medicines dispensed.
3   The pharmacy must record any advice given, interventions made and referrals, where the pharmacist judges this to be clinically appropriate.

Q7 The essential service 'promoting healthy lifestyles' includes offering opportunistic advice to the following when a prescription is presented. A community pharmacist would offer advice to:

1   Patients with asthma
2   Patients who smoke
3   Patients with high blood pressure

Q8 Which of the following statements about clinical effectiveness is (are) correct?

1   Clinical effectiveness is the same as clinical governance.
2   Accurate records of clinical audit are needed to demonstrate clinical effectiveness.
3   Pharmacists can contribute to the clinical effectiveness of prescribing through the MUR service.

Directions for questions 9 and 10: the following questions consist of a statement in the left-hand column followed by a second statement in the right-hand column.
Decide whether the first statement is true or false.
Decide whether the second statement is true or false.
Then choose:

A   if both statements are true and the second statement is a correct explanation of the first statement
B   if both statements are true but the second statement is NOT a correct explanation of the first statement
C   if the first statement is true but the second statement is false
D   if the first statement is false but the second statement is true
E   if both statements are false

Directions summarised:

A:	True	True	second statement is **a correct explanation** of the first
B:	True	True	second statement is **NOT a correct explanation** of the first
C:	True	False	
D:	False	True	
E:	False	False	

Q9

- *Statement 1*: Out-of-date spironolactone tablets removed from the dispensary cannot be disposed of with out-of-date ibuprofen 400 mg tablets (pack size 24) from the stock room.
- *Statement 2*: The special waste regulations 1996 specify that different categories of waste cannot be mixed.

Q10

- *Statement 1*: A monitored dosage system should be offered to all elderly people requesting this service.
- *Statement 2*: Under the Disability Discrimination Act 1995, pharmacists providing services in the UK have a legal obligation to make reasonable adjustments to their services.

Case studies

Level 1

Tamara is a third-year pharmacy undergraduate who is part of an inter-professional group of four students. The other students in her group are studying medicine, nursing and social work. The tutor has asked each student to talk informally to the rest of their group about their profession and how it may relate to other professional groups.

- Prepare a brief summary for Tamara, using bullet points, of how the contractual framework for community pharmacy can relate to GPs, nurses and social workers.

Level 2

Ryan is a preregistration trainee who is only in the first few weeks of his training. He is enjoying his work but had a difficult incident today when handing out a prescription. The customer asked him if she could have her tablets in weekly blister packs as she is a bit forgetful and finds it hard to remember to take her tablets. She also said that she has difficulties with her hands and finds the glass medicine bottles far too heavy to handle. Ryan asked the dispensary team if this was possible. They were very dismissive as they were extremely busy at the time and the relief pharmacist was on the telephone. He decided to show some initiative and told the customer that it would not be possible. She started to become angry and upset and said she would be making a formal complaint. Ryan came into work early the following morning as he wanted to discuss the incident with his tutor.

The preregistration tutor asks Ryan to think about the following areas:

- what are the issues involved in this case?
- what could Ryan have done differently?
- what preregistration performance standards could this incident relate to?

Level 3

Ben has completed the second year of his pharmacy degree course and is pleased to have been offered a 4-week summer placement in his local community pharmacy. He has not worked in community pharmacy before and is looking forward to the opportunity to gain some experience. On his first day he is disappointed to find that the regular pharmacist he arranged the placement with, has just started his 3-week holiday. The senior assistant seems quite distracted and appears only vaguely aware that Ben is due to start work today. One member of staff has called in sick and the locum pharmacist arrives only one minute before opening time.

Ben is quickly assigned to the prescription reception area and the process of receiving and handing out prescriptions is hurriedly explained. He is also instructed to shadow the staff on the medicines counter and help to fill some shelves as there is a large section of remerchandising taking place.

The morning proceeds quite quickly and Ben is keen to learn from his experience. His first impression is that the pharmacy seems quite disorganised. He decides to keep a diary record of some of the main events of the day.

Extracts from Ben's diary – Day 1

- A customer asked me some questions about prescription-collection and delivery services. I was unsure how to answer his questions so I asked the pharmacist and dispensing assistant. The dispensing assistant spoke to the customer briefly and I listened to their conversation. My impression is that the staff did not seem particularly helpful to the customer.

- An elderly man got quite upset with me because he said I had given him the wrong tablets as he had misheard me when I asked for his name. The pharmacist managed to sort it out but it caused quite a big problem at the time. The pharmacist reassured me that I was not to blame. I kept thinking about why it had happened but everyone seemed too busy to take much interest in the details
- A customer had a repeat prescription that she leaves in the pharmacy without seeing her doctor. It seemed to take the dispensing assistant a long time to find the prescription. The customer then had to come back to collect her medication.
- In the afternoon I was left on the medicines counter on my own as the other staff were busy completing a new display of holiday healthcare products. I did not feel at all comfortable and was embarrassed to keep asking the pharmacist questions.

- Identify the clinical governance issues in this case study.

References

1   Department of Health. *Pharmacy in the Future: implementing the NHS Plan. A programme for pharmacy in the NHS.* London: Department of Health, 2000. www.dh.gov.uk/en/Publicationsandstatistics/Publications/PublicationsPolicyAndGuidance/Browsable/DH_4098182 (accessed 5 September 2007).

2   Department of Health. *Spending Review 2004 Public Service Agreement.* London: Department of Health, 2004. www.dh.gov.uk/en/Aboutus/HowDHworks/Servicestandardsandcommitments/DHPublicServiceAgreement/DH_4106188 (accessed 11 September 2007).

3   News item. Bulk of enhanced services made up of four types. *Pharm J* 2006; **277**: 628.

4   Pharmaceutical Services Negotiating Committee. *NHS Community Pharmacy Contractual Framework. Essential Service – Dispensing.* www.psnc.org.uk/uploaded_txt/Service%20Spec%20ES1%20%20Dispensing%20_v1%2010%20Oct%2004_.pdf (accessed 5 September 2007).

5   Centre for Pharmacy Postgraduate Education. *Distance Learning Pack: repeat dispensing from pathfinder to practice.* Manchester: Centre for Pharmacy Postgraduate Education.

6   Welsh Centre for Pharmacy Postgraduate Education. *Distance Learning Pack: repeat dispensing arrangements in Wales.* Cardiff: Welsh Centre for Pharmacy Postgraduate Education.

7   Pharmaceutical Services Negotiating Committee. *NHS Community Pharmacy Contractual Framework. Essential Service – Repeat Dispensing.* www.psnc.org.uk/uploaded_txt/Service%20Spec%20ES2%20%20Repeat%20dispensing%20_v1%2010%20Oct%2004_.pdf (accessed 5 September 2007).

8   Royal Pharmaceutical Society of Great Britain. *The Hazardous Waste Regulations (England and Wales) 2005 and Information for Scotland. Interim practice guidance for community pharmacists.* www.rpsgb.org.uk/pdfs/ hazwastecommphguid.pdf_(accessed 5 September 2007).

9   Department of Health. *Choosing Health: making healthy choices easier.* London: Department of Health, 2005. www.dh.gov.uk/en/Publications andstatistics/Publications/PublicationsPolicyAndGuidance/Browsable/ DH_4097491 (accessed 5 September 2007).

10   Department of Health. *Choosing Health Through Pharmacy. A programme for pharmaceutical public health 2005–2015.* London: Department of Health, 2005. www.dh.gov.uk/en/Publicationsandstatistics/ Publications/ PublicationsPolicyAndGuidance/DH_4107494 (accessed 5 September 2007).

11   Pharmaceutical Services Negotiating Committee. *NHS Community Pharmacy Contractual Framework. Essential Service – Support for Self-care.* www.psnc.org.uk/uploaded_txt/Service%20spec%20ES6%20-%20 Support%20for%20self-care%20_v1%2010%20Oct%2004_.pdf (accessed 5 September).

12   Royal Pharmaceutical Society of Great Britain. Practice and Quality Improvement Directorate. *Pharm J* 2005; **275**: 203–204.

13   Royal Pharmaceutical Society of Great Britain. *Medicines Ethics and Practice (30).* Practice guidance 4.3.30. London: Royal Pharmaceutical Society of Great Britain, 2006.

14   Royal Pharmaceutical Society of Great Britain. Guidance document. Consultation on SOPs for dispensing. *Pharm J* 2001; **266**: 616–619.

15   News feature. Writing SOPs, where should you start? *Pharm J* 2003; **271**: 443–444.

16   Royal Pharmaceutical Society of Great Britain. *Developing and Implementing SOPs for Dispensing.* London: Royal Pharmaceutical Society of Great Britain, 2001. www.rpsgb.org.uk/pdfs/sops.pdf (accessed 5 September 2007).

17   NHS Primary Care Contracting. *Community Pharmacy Assurance Framework.* www.primarycarecontracting.nhs.uk/114.php (accessed 5 September 2007).

18   Pharmaceutical Services Negotiating Committee. *New Contract Workbook 2005–2006.* www.psnc.org.uk/uploaded_txt/WORKBOOK %20-%20FINAL%20VERSION.pdf (accessed 5 September 2007).

19   Department of Health. *Pharmacy Contract: non compliance and dispute resolution.* http://www.primarycarecontracting.nhs.uk/uploads/ Pharmacy/jul06_uploads/noncompliance_and_dispute_resolution.pdf (accessed 5 September 2007).

20   Disability Discrimination Act 1995. www.opsi.gov.uk/acts/acts1995/ 1995050.htm (accessed 5 September 2007).

21   Pharmaceutical Services Negotiating Committee. *Pharmacy and the Disability Discrimination Act.* www.psnc.org.uk/index.php?type= page&pid=93&k=4 (accessed 10 May 2007).

22   Rosenbloom K, Wakeman R, Scrimshaw. The Disability Discrimination Act. *Pharm J* 2005; **275**: 747–750.

23   Department of Health. *Drug Tariff* (published monthly) Part VIA. London: Department of Health.

24   NHS Primary Care Contracting. *Disability Discrimination Act – A Resource Kit*. www.primarycarecontracting.nhs.uk/98.php (accessed 5 September 2007).

25   Bellingham C. Introducing the new Scottish contract. *Pharm J* 2005; **275**: 637.

26   Scottish Executive. *Delivering for Health*.   www.scotland.gov.uk/Publications/2005/11/02102635/26360 (accessed 5 September 2007).

Further information

Royal Pharmaceutical Society of Great Britain. *National Resources Available to Support the Community Pharmacy Contract (England and Wales)*. www.rpsgb.org/pdfs/cpcontractnatresources.pdf (accessed 5 September 2007).

5

Medicines use review

Community pharmacy will need to make changes in order to provide the services that patients and the new NHS want and need.
(A Vision for Pharmacy in the New NHS, Department of Health[1])

Checkpoint

Before reading on, think about the following questions to identify your own knowledge gaps in this area:

- What is the main purpose of a medicines use review (MUR)?
- How does an MUR differ from a prescription intervention (PI) service?
- What are the requirements to become accredited to offer an MUR service?
- Describe how suitable patients can be identified for an MUR.

Advanced services form the second tier of the national contract. Medicines use review (MUR) and prescription intervention (PI) were the first advanced services to be introduced. These services are considered together as they both involve a review of medicines usage. An MUR is planned in advance and is undertaken regularly. A PI service is unplanned and is initiated as a result of a prescription that has significant medication issues that need to be discussed in more detail. The provision of these advanced services involves accreditation of both the pharmacist and the premises. The community pharmacist has always been involved in the review of medicines usage on an informal basis. The introduction of this advanced service is significant, as this is the first time that community pharmacists have been involved in a nationally recognised and remunerated clinical review service.

There has been some confusion about the purpose and limitations of the MUR service. The MUR is essentially a compliance and concordance review that aims to help people use their medicines more effectively. It involves identifying problems with medicines, providing advice and suggesting changes to the general practitioner (GP). The MUR is not intended to be a full level 3 medication review and the pharmacist does not have access to the patient's notes and test results. Initially an MUR looks at the patient's compliance with taking medicines as directed by the prescriber. The pharmacist can then make recommendations to the patient, carer or other healthcare professionals to improve compliance and reduce drug-related problems.

The initial participation of pharmacists in offering this advanced service was significantly below the anticipated 200 MURs per pharmacy by April 2006.[2] Some of the reasons suggested for the lack of involvement in this essential service are:

- lack of acceptance of this new service by both the patient and the GP
- confusion about the amount of time required to conduct an MUR
- lack of pharmacy resources in terms of both staff and time
- problems with the provision of a suitable consultation area
- the paperwork and record keeping involved in the process is overly complicated.

Potentially the offering of an MUR and PI service will benefit patients and lead to improved pharmaceutical care. Involvement in this service is also rewarding for the pharmacist both professionally and financially. This chapter aims to offer a practical guide to offering a MUR service in the pharmacy.

Accreditation

As a quality-assurance mechanism both the pharmacy premises and the pharmacist need to be accredited to offer an advanced service. The essential requirements for offering an MUR service are outlined in Box 5.1.

Box 5.1   Accreditation of pharmacist and premises for an MUR service

---

- Premises must have a consultation area that:
  - is clearly designated and distinct from the general area of the pharmacy
  - allows the pharmacist and the customer to sit down together
  - is somewhere that they can talk at normal volumes without being overheard by staff and customers.
- The pharmacist must have:
  - an MUR certificate from a relevant higher education institute
  - sent the certificate to the appropriate primary care organisation
  - complied with the clinical governance requirements under the new contract.

Pharmacist accreditation

A competence-based framework has been developed for the assessment of pharmacists providing the MUR service.[3] The framework is not designed to be an exhaustive list of competencies but includes key elements that can be subject to reliable assessment. Higher education institutions (HEIs) will make arrangements for the assessment of pharmacists within this framework. Individual HEIs will approach the competency framework in different ways and have different methods of assessment. Universities offering this assessment as higher education providers have quality-assurance processes in place for learning and assessment. For consistency there will be no accreditation of prior learning, and all pharmacists wishing to become accredited will need to pass the assessment. There are five competencies and each competency is linked to a number of behavioural statements. The competency framework is summarised in Table 5.1.

Table 5.1 Main competencies for accreditation of pharmacists to deliver an MUR service

Main area	Specific competencies
Clinical and pharmaceutical knowledge	1 Demonstrate relevant clinical and pharmaceutical knowledge to deliver MUR, taking into account the patient's individual needs 2 Demonstrate the ability to identify and make recommendations around therapeutic issues relating to patient safety and clinical and cost-effectiveness
Accessing and applying information	3 Demonstrate the ability to identify, access, evaluate and use available written sources of information 4 Demonstrate the ability to reach a shared agreement with patients
Documentation and referral	5 Ensure recommendations agreed with the patient are documented and appropriately communicated in a timely manner

There are a number of training options to choose from depending on the pharmacist's preferred learning method, and their prior knowledge and experience. Some pharmacists may wish to update their clinical skills and knowledge before undergoing the assessment. In some cases this may be inappropriate and the pharmacist will be ready to undertake the competence-based assessment without any additional training. Choices of online and paper-based assessment methods are available. Some HEIs that offer postgraduate clinical programmes such as diplomas have integrated the competency-based assessment into their existing postgraduate courses. Further details of training and assessment for offering an MUR service are available on the Pharmaceutical Services Negotiating Committee (PSNC) website.[4]

Premises accreditation

One of the common criticisms of community pharmacy premises by both customers and patient groups is their lack of privacy. A study evaluating NHS Direct referrals to community pharmacies noted that lack of privacy was of some concern to patients.[5] The introduction of consultation rooms has been a positive step in addressing this issue. Under the current terms, the provision of a consultation room is not a requirement if the contractor is only aiming to provide essential services. However, if the pharmacist wishes to deliver an MUR service then the installation of a consultation room is essential. In the majority of cases the MUR will be carried out face to face with the patient in the pharmacy consultation room. If a pharmacist wishes to provide the MUR service in another location, for example in a patient's home or in a day care centre, application must be made to the primary care trust (PCT) using standard documentation.[6]

The three requirements of the pharmacy consultation room for the purposes of delivering an MUR service are clearly stated in the service specification,[7] and summarised in Box 5.1. The specification is deliberately loose to allow contractors to work within the physical limitations of their individual pharmacies.

Guidance on how to make space for a new consultation room has appeared in the *Pharmaceutical Journal*.[8] If a pharmacy is planning a new consultation room the main issues to consider are:

- the provision of adequate space from the beginning
- meeting the needs of pharmacists and customers
- future proofing for new services or technology
- compensating for any lost retail sales space.

There is no minimum or maximum size for the room specified but the requirement for at least two people to be able to sit down will influence the size of the room. In addition the Disability Discrimination Act will need to be taken into account when considering ease of access into the room. The room needs to be sited in a suitable location. For example, if the room is installed between the medicines counter and the dispensary this can interrupt the natural flow of work in this busy area of the pharmacy. For the purpose of offering an MUR service the room requires very little equipment. The main resources required are a seating area for two people, a suitable table or desk and the appropriate storage of recording forms, reference materials and information leaflets. To future-proof the room it is necessary to consider how the room will be used to fulfil future advanced and enhanced services. Examples of areas to be considered above the basic specification include:

- the installation of a networked computer to access patient records and make electronic records
- the facility to print information for use by the patient and the pharmacist
- storage facilities for diagnostic-testing equipment and consumables
- secure filing facilities for paper records
- the safe disposal of clinical waste
- access to hot and cold water and waste disposal
- a suitable number of electrical power points for any equipment.

Unless the pharmacy has a suitable under-utilised area of stock room or other non-sales area, there will be a loss of retail sales space. The design and integration of the room into the pharmacy therefore needs specialist planning to minimise the impact this will have on sales.

The final stage of the accreditation process is the completion of a self-certification form.[9] The pharmacist makes a declaration that:

- there is an acceptable system of clinical governance
- patients will be recruited to the MUR service in line with local PCT patient group priorities
- the consultation room complies with the service specification.

The completed form and a copy of the pharmacist's accreditation certificate are sent to the PCT.

Planning the MUR service

Once accredited, the pharmacist needs to consider a number of practical issues before being able to deliver the MUR service.

Identification of suitable patients

To identify suitable patients the pharmacist must ensure that the patient is included in the MUR service specification criteria. The following conditions need to be satisfied:

- a patient on multiple medicines and those with long-term conditions
- the MUR can be conducted every 12 months provided the patient has been using the pharmacy for the dispensing of prescriptions for the previous 3 months. This is to ensure the pharmacist has a certain basic amount of information on the patient on the patient medication record (PMR) system
- a pharmacist can accept requests from patients for an MUR or referrals from other healthcare professionals provided the above two criteria are met
- the primary care organisation (PCO) may identify specific patient groups that would be appropriate to target, based on the needs of the local health economy. For example a PCO may prioritise ischaemic heart disease, stroke, diabetes or mental health patients
- an MUR can be undertaken when a significant problem presents during the dispensing of a prescription. This PI is over and above the basic interventions that make up the essential dispensing service. In this case the patient would not have to meet the first two criteria stated.

Promotion and marketing of the service

There are a number of promotional materials available, to help the pharmacist communicate the benefits of this service and emphasise that this service is free to the patient. It is important that the promotional material is accurate and professional in appearance. The key message on any promotional material is that the MUR is a one-to-one discussion with the pharmacist on how to get the most out of medicines being taken. Examples of suitable material are available on the PSNC website.[10] The use of printed material needs to be reinforced by a personal approach to specific patients who would benefit from this service. Many pharmacists use the opportunity to promote the MUR service when handing out repeat medication. In some cases an MUR can result from a patient query about their medication at the point of dispensing. The query can result in the pharmacist inviting the patient to attend for an MUR, for a more detailed discussion about their medicines.

An alternative approach is for the pharmacist to identify specific patient groups. For example the pharmacist may use their PMRs to identify patients with diabetes. Diabetes UK supports the community pharmacy contract and recognises the benefit of improved access to medicines-management information and advice. An article promoting the benefits of the MUR service appeared in the Diabetes UK patient publication *Balance* magazine.[11]

Other examples of taking a proactive approach include the identification of patients with specific characteristics or patients taking certain medication: Examples include:

- patients over 75 years taking more than four medicines

- patients who have frequent falls
- asthma patients that are under 18 years old
- patients taking proton pump inhibitors
- patients taking benzodiazepines or the 'z drugs' (zopiclone, zolpidem and zaleplon).

For the MUR service to be marketed effectively it is necessary to present a coherent message from all members of the pharmacy team. This will involve a detailed briefing of all of the team members who have regular contact with patients.

Communication with the patient's GP

The introduction of a successful MUR service is dependent on clear communication with local GP practices. The pharmacist should aim to speak to local GPs about the rationale of the MUR service and what it aims to achieve. Ideally this communication should take the form of a short presentation to the local GP practice meeting. This preferred method encourages dialogue and discussion about the benefits of the MUR process and fosters closer working relationships. If a presentation is not possible, the use of a briefing paper including contact details is another option. Any briefing material that is circulated to GP practices should emphasise the purpose of an MUR.[12]

The main purpose of an MUR is to identify:

- if the patient uses their medicine as prescribed
- if the patient understands how to use their medicine
- any issues affecting the correct use of medicine
- if the patient knows why their medicines have been prescribed
- any side-effects
- medicines that are no longer used.

Any communication with GPs should make it clear that an MUR does *not* include any discussion of:

- changes to drug treatment
- a medical condition beyond its drug treatment
- the effectiveness of treatment based on test results.

When discussing MURs with local GPs, it is useful to discuss how the results of the MUR are communicated and if there are ways of working more closely with the practice. For example, some pharmacists liaise with their local practices to ensure that the timing of an MUR does not clash with a full regular medication review at the surgery. This is an excellent opportunity to work more closely with the practice pharmacist and ensure that a positive message about this service is communicated. It is recognised by some PCOs that MURs can contribute to the Quality and Outcomes Framework (QOF) of the GMS contract.[13] While it is accepted that an MUR is not the same as a medication review as defined in national documentation,[14] it can contribute considerably to the medication review process. For some groups of patients, such as those being prescribed four or more repeat medicines, a medication review is included in the QOF. The recording of significant lifestyle advice for specific patients is also a potential area where the MUR documentation can provide useful evidence for the medical practice.

Access to resources during the MUR

Before performing the first MUR some thought needs to be given to how the pharmacist will access resources during the consultation. Areas to be considered include:

- access to the PMR in the consultation area. If the PMR is not linked to this area then a copy of the patient record will need to be printed off in advance of the consultation
- reference sources
- patient information leaflets (including lifestyle and health-promotion information)
- signposting information
- placebo devices that may be needed for demonstration purposes
- the MUR form.

As the MUR is usually booked on an appointment basis, there may be the opportunity for the pharmacist to check the patient profile before the MUR and ensure that appropriate supporting information will be available in the consultation room.

Planning appointments

To offer this service the pharmacist will be based in the consultation room and will not be in direct contact with the dispensing area. This has implications for the supervision of dispensing and sales of medicines. The Royal Pharmaceutical Society of Great Britain (RPSGB) interim guidance states that pharmacy medicines may be sold and prescriptions that have been checked for clinical appropriateness and accuracy may be supplied, provided that robust standard operating procedures (SOPs) are in place.[15] This means that each prescription must have been checked by the pharmacist before it can be dispensed. It would therefore be impractical to have several MUR appointments arranged during a busy dispensing period. However, it may be possible to conduct isolated MURs during quieter dispensing periods. There is some discussion about the length of time an MUR should take. The time taken will impact on the quality of the service and the level of remuneration for the time invested. At present there are no specific guidelines on how long an MUR should take. In practice there is a wide variation in the time taken to carry out a review. The time taken may range from a few minutes to nearly an hour depending on the type of presenting patient. To offer a service that is meaningful and include time for relevant discussion and recording of outcomes, an allocated 15 minute minimum time slot would seem realistic. Some pharmacists prefer to absorb these appointments into the quieter dispensing periods. Another option is the employment of a locum pharmacist to provide additional cover. However, this has practical cost implications, especially if the booked patients do not attend their appointment. The non-attendance of patients for their scheduled MUR appointment has significant implications on the effective running of the pharmacy.[16]

One practical system is to identify periods of the week where the regular dispensing workload is likely to be less. For example it is useful to find out the number of GPs attending morning and afternoon surgery and details of any regular training sessions where the surgery is closed for a short period. It is also beneficial to have an overall profile of the dispensing workload on a daily and weekly basis. Potential 30 minute slots can then be marked in the diary and offered as MUR appointments. Use of appointment cards and a reminder phone call on the morning of the appointment can help to reduce the number of non-attendances.

Conducting an MUR

Having considered some preliminary practical issues, this section considers how to conduct an MUR and breaks down the process into stages. An example of a completed MUR form is provided in Appendix 1, p. 274).

The stages involved in conducting an MUR are outlined in Figure 5.1.

Meeting the patient

On meeting the patient, the pharmacist should introduce themselves. If the patient is unknown to the pharmacist, their identity should be established. Before starting the MUR, put the patient at ease and pay attention to their comfort and privacy. The overall purpose of the MUR should be briefly explained and the patient provided with some indication of the length of time available for the consultation.

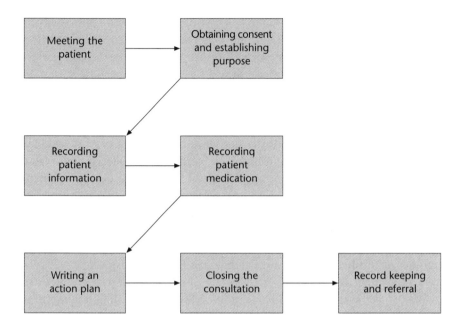

Figure 5.1 The stages involved in conducting a medicines use review.

Obtaining consent and establishing purpose

Before the MUR can commence it should be established that the patient has:

- received information on the MUR and consented to the review process
- agreed that information may be shared with their GP
- agreed that information may be shared with others such as carers. If the patient wishes for the information to be shared with others they must specify their names.

The patient should also be asked what they hope to get out of the review. For example they may wish to learn more about their medication in general or have specific queries about certain aspects of their medication. All of this information is recorded on the MUR form.

Recording patient information

The first page of the standard MUR form is to record identification information for the patient, the GP and the pharmacy. The section on basic health data is designed to be brief and should not contain elaborate details. As this is not a full medication review it is clear that the pharmacist does not have access to medical records and test results and is consequently working with information provided by the patient. However there is a lot of vital information that can be recorded that will help the pharmacist when making recommendations. The main areas of discussion should focus on:

- significant previous adverse drug reactions
- medical history as described by the patient
- known allergies and sensitivities
- monitoring as described by the patient and recorded in the PMR.

It is appropriate in this section to ask some leading questions about lifestyle factors such as smoking, alcohol intake and dietary habits.

Recording patient medication

The centre of the form consists of a list of the patient's medication and the dosage regimen. Some PMR systems have the capability to electronically transfer the PMR directly across to this part of the form. The dosage of the medication as the patient takes it should be recorded along with a brief statement of the patient's knowledge of the medicines use. The next stage is to determine how compliant the patient is with their medication. This is assessed as: always, frequent, seldom or never. The appropriateness of the formulation and an indication if the medicine is working is also recorded. The patient is asked if they experience any side-effects, and brief details are recorded. The final part of this section of the MUR form is to record a general comment next to each medicine. The purpose of this comment is to clarify to the patient why the medicine is being taken. For example: losartan 50 mg tablets 'causes blood vessels to relax and so lowers blood pressure'. The recording of medication should also include any medication that has been purchased over the counter and why it is being used. For example: 'senna tablets purchased for constipation as this is not being eased by prescribed lactulose'.

Writing an action plan

When considering writing the action plan, three factors need to be applied to each medicine:

- appropriateness in terms of indication and also to eliminate any potentially unnecessary medication. For example co-codamol being used in addition to paracetamol
- safety issues with respect to side-effects, drug interactions and contraindications. For example if there is indication of muscle pain with a statin this would need to be highlighted in the document
- effectiveness of the medicine when considering the choice, dose,

formulation, non-compliance and monitoring. For example a patient may be struggling to use a standard monitored dose inhaler and may benefit from the use of a breath actuated inhaler.

The purpose of this summary section is to record information that is useful to both the patient and the GP, however straightforward this may seem. A record of any lifestyle advice given or signposting to another service should be recorded. The GP will find updated information such as smoking status and body mass index (BMI) useful. The action plan consists of usually up to four action points that are prioritised and allocated to the patient, the pharmacist or the GP.

Closing the consultation

At the end of the MUR each recommendation of the proposed action plan should be discussed with the patient. The next stage should be discussed, which may include making an appointment to see the GP within a specified time period.

Record keeping and referral

The standard form for the Community Pharmacy Medicines Use Review and Prescription Intervention Service can be completed manually or electronically.[17] Ideally the form should be filled in electronically as this allows amendments to be made and provides a much clearer record of the MUR. A badly written handwritten form can create a poor impression to both the patient and the GP. Handwritten forms are scanned into the patient's record at the surgery so need to be clear and legible.

A copy of both the MUR summary and the recommendations will be given to the patient for information. A summary of any recommendations will be sent to the patient's GP. A record of the MUR will be made on the patient's PMR record.

When recording summary information for the GP, check that the statement is both useful and relevant.

Top tips on providing MUR summary information for GPs

- It is not helpful for the GP to receive a summary form for all their patients with diabetes that states: 'Check regular blood glucose monitoring'. However, if during the course of the MUR a general

$\rightarrow$

lack of regular blood glucose monitoring was revealed, the pharmacist should try and find the reason for this and make a record on the form. For example: 'Patient not taking many readings as finds difficulty in using blood glucose meter. Demonstrated meter and patient now appears confident to use more regularly. Refer to practice nurse if problem persists'.

■ Most blood monitoring tests such as renal function and electrolytes with angiotensin-converting enzyme (ACE) inhibitors will be arranged routinely by the GP practice. Only recommend these monitoring tests if the patient has no recollection of being monitored.

■ The changes suggested to a prescriber may include issues such as:
  – lack of adequate dosage instructions
  – unwanted medicines
  – changes to dosage form
  – generic substitutions for branded items
  – dose optimisation to avoid multiple doses of a lower strength
  – clinical effectiveness issues that have been highlighted by the local PCO, for example highlighting a patient that is on a treatment rather than a maintenance dose of a proton pump inhibitor.

Consultation skills

For many pharmacists, sitting down with a patient in a consultation room is a new experience. The skill set required is very different from patient counselling or responding to symptoms. During the early stages of offering a MUR service it is useful to reflect on which areas of the process are performed well and which areas need to be highlighted for future continuing professional development (CPD) activity.

Practical solutions to patient problems

Many of the problems encountered during an MUR consultation are of a practical nature and the pharmacist is ideally placed to offer possible solutions or make referrals.

The main areas of patient need are usually:

■ access to medicines
■ intentional compliance issues
■ non-intentional compliance issues
■ clinical issues surrounding medication.

Access to medicines

The patient may have synchronisation problems with their repeat prescription or problems ordering their repeat medication. There may be issues of mobility and the patient is dependent on carers for obtaining their repeat prescription. The pharmacist can discuss practical ways of improving access to medicines such as prescription-collection and delivery services.

Intentional compliance issues

In some cases the patient may lack motivation in the management of their medicines or have concerns over possible side-effects or believe their medication is not effective. This may result in the patient not taking the medication as intended and this should be highlighted as part of the MUR process.

Non-intentional compliance issues

Non-intentional compliance issues can be caused by a wide range of patient needs and these areas need to be explored carefully. Some common examples of non-intentional compliance and possible practical solutions are summarised in Table 5.2. Before suggesting the use of a compliance aid, the first step is always to see if the medication regimen can be simplified in any way. For example, it may be possible for the patient to be prescribed a long-acting preparation to reduce the number of doses. The use of aids such as reminder charts, colour coding, setting alarm clocks and prominent posters may be sufficient to solve some compliance problems. If a compliance aid is required there is a useful list of companies to contact in the further resources section at the end of this chapter.

Clinical issues surrounding medication

A useful overview of some practical hints and tips when conducting an MUR for different types of patient is provided in Figure 5.2.

Two common clinical issues that need to be explored during an MUR include:

- side-effects resulting in the patient no longer taking their medication
- the medication is no longer controlling their symptoms, resulting in the purchase of additional medicines such as painkillers.

Table 5.2 Non-intentional compliance issues and possible practical solutions

Compliance issue	Possible solution
Difficulty in using a product form such as an inhaler device, topical preparation or eye drops	Offer to demonstrate device and offer support Consider whether an alternative form may be more appropriate
Inaccurate measurement of liquid doses	Demonstration of accurate dosage measurement
Manual dexterity problems due to arthritis, stroke, tremor or muscle weakness and is unable to open child-resistant containers	Consider use of non-child-resistant containers
Memory problems and/or confusion. The patient finds it difficult to cope with a complex medication regimen	Consider compliance aids such as monitored dose community blister packs, dosette boxes, reminder charts Involvement of carer in administration of medication
Swallowing difficulties	Discuss other options and change to liquid formulations if available
Unable to understand directions or the directions are not clear such as 'as directed' labelling	Ensure labelling is specific and spend time clarifying dosage instructions

All clinical issues should be recorded and referred. In more complex cases a full medication review should be recommended.

Summary

A SWOT analysis (strengths, weaknesses, opportunities and threats) of MURs was undertaken by five groups of pharmacists attending MUR workshops run by the University of Reading.[18] The weaknesses were identified as:

- service requires investment of time and resources
- paper-based service at present
- no access to patient records
- lack of GP and patient awareness
- restrictions on numbers of MURs that can be completed
- may be unable to meet patient expectations
- housebound patients may not be able to access the service.

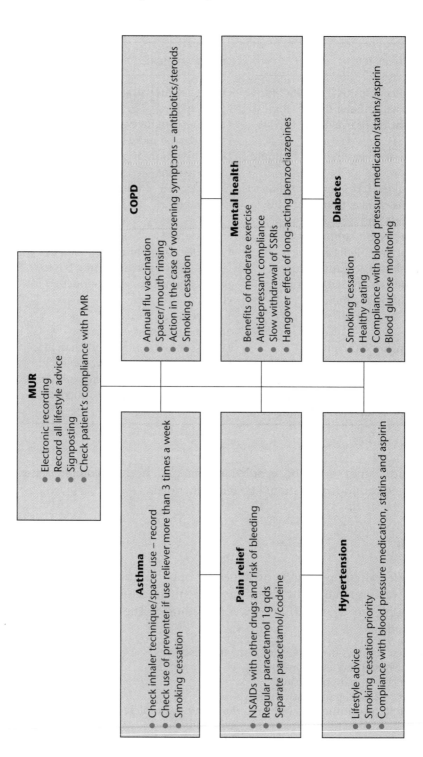

MUR
- Electronic recording
- Record all lifestyle advice
- Signposting
- Check patient's compliance with PMR

COPD
- Annual flu vaccination
- Spacer/mouth rinsing
- Action in the case of worsening symptoms – antibiotics/steroids
- Smoking cessation

Mental health
- Benefits of moderate exercise
- Antidepressant compliance
- Slow withdrawal of SSRIs
- Hangover effect of long-acting benzodiazepines

Diabetes
- Smoking cessation
- Healthy eating
- Compliance with blood pressure medication/statins/aspirin
- Blood glucose monitoring

Asthma
- Check inhaler technique/spacer use – record
- Check use of preventer if use reliever more than 3 times a week
- Smoking cessation

Pain relief
- NSAIDs with other drugs and risk of bleeding
- Regular paracetamol 1 g qds
- Separate paracetamol/codeine

Hypertension
- Lifestyle advice
- Smoking cessation priority
- Compliance with blood pressure medication, statins and aspirin

Figure 5.2 Selected hints and tips for conducting a medicines use review for patients with different conditions. COPD, chronic obstructive pulmonary disease; NSAID, non-steroidal anti-inflammatory drug; SSRI, selective serotonin reuptake inhibitor.

The main areas of weakness when delivering this advanced service are the practical use of time and resources. The issue of time management and integration of this service into the pharmacy working day are significant issues for this service to be successful.

Top tips for time management when delivering an MUR service

- Train members of the dispensing team who are speaking directly to patients to promote the service.
- Identify potentially quieter periods for MUR appointment slots.
- Delegate the initial groundwork to a suitably trained pharmacy technician, for example collecting patient data for the first part of the form and also collating relevant information from the PMR
- Prepare for the MUR by looking at the PMR and make a note of any particular areas that need to be explored in more detail.
- Ensure that the patient is aware of the purpose of the MUR and recognises that there is a time constraint on the consultation.
- Immediately after the MUR, process the paperwork and make a note on the PMR.

During the first year of implementation the uptake of the MUR service accounted for only a small proportion of allocated funding.[19] There is a wide variation between PCOs in the level of MUR provision. At the time of writing there are signs of growth in the number of contractors claiming payment for MURs and the number of MURs performed in each pharmacy.[20] The service is starting to become more established and pharmacists are using many different strategies to promote and deliver this unique service. The successful delivery of this clinical advanced service is dependent on well-developed time-management skills and the full support of the entire pharmacy team.

Implications for practice

Activity 1

Devise a template to self-assess your consultation skills when conducting an MUR.

- Are there any CPD needs that are highlighted as a result of this exercise?

Activity 2

- What are your local PCT priorities for MURs?
- How can you identify specific patient groups using your PMR system?
- Assess the marketing material available for promoting MURs. Can any of this material be adapted to provide a more specific local message?

Multiple choice questions

Directions for questions 1 and 2: each of the questions or incomplete statements in this section is followed by five suggested answers. Select the best answer in each case.

Q1 Which of the following patients would definitely *not* be a suitable candidate for a medicines use review?

A   A patient taking atorvastatin, aspirin and ramipril and using a salbutamol inhaler
B   An asthmatic patient who has been referred by the asthma nurse at the local surgery
C   A patient with acute sinusitis who has been prescribed amoxicillin
D   A teenager on two types of anti-epileptic medication
E   An elderly patient who is housebound and on a number of regular repeat medications

Q2 Which of the following best describes the purpose of an MUR?

A   The provision and recording of specific lifestyle advice for patients
B   A clinical review of all medication being taken by the patient
C   A discussion of a patient's drug treatment based on their knowledge of their test results
D   A consultation based on compliance and concordance
E   An opportunity for the patient to discuss medical problems with another healthcare professional

Directions for questions 3 to 5: for each numbered question select the one lettered option above it which is most closely related to it. Within each group of questions each lettered option may be used once, more than once, or not at all.

The following options all relate to different issues that may arise during an MUR.

A   Compliance
B   Concordance
C   Clinical effectiveness

D   Patient safety
E   Inappropriate dose

Select from A to E which one of the above fits the following statements

Q3   A patient has been prescribed omeprazole 40 mg capsules, once daily for a duodenal ulcer. On questioning the patient you find out that they are taking the medication regularly and the PMR indicates that they have been supplied with this medication for the past 4 months.
Q4   A patient is taking simvastatin 40 mg tablets regularly once daily in the evening and has no knowledge of why the medicine has been prescribed.
Q5   A young adult patient with diabetes reveals that sometimes they miss doses of insulin at the weekend as they are often busy.

Directions for questions 6 to 8: each of the questions or incomplete statements in this section is followed by three responses. For each question ONE or MORE of the responses is (are) correct. Decide which of the responses is (are) correct. Then choose:

A   if 1, 2 and 3 are correct
B   if 1 and 2 only are correct
C   if 2 and 3 only are correct
D   if 1 only is correct
E   if 3 only is correct

Directions summarised:
A: 1, 2, 3   B: 1, 2 only   C: 2, 3 only   D: 1 only   E: 3 only

Q6   A consultation room for a community pharmacy must satisfy the following criteria:

1   The room is clearly designated and distinct from the general area of the pharmacy
2   The room is completely soundproof
3   There is space for a minimum of three people

Q7   To become accredited to offer an MUR service a pharmacist must:

1   Hold a postgraduate clinical pharmacy qualification
2   Carry out a number of practice MURs before being certified to offer the service
3   Hold an MUR certificate from a relevant higher education institute

Q8   To commence the provision of an MUR service the pharmacist needs to confirm the following information with the local PCT:

1   Patients will be recruited to the MUR service in line with local PCT patient group priorities
2   The consultation room complies with the service specification
3   There is an acceptable system of clinical governance

Directions for questions 9 and 10: The following questions consist of a statement in the left-hand column followed by a second statement in the right-hand column.
Decide whether the first statement is true or false.
Decide whether the second statement is true or false.
Then choose:

A   if both statements are true and the second statement is a correct explanation of the first statement
B   if both statements are true but the second statement is NOT a correct explanation of the first statement
C   if the first statement is true but the second statement is false
D   if the first statement is false but the second statement is true
E   if both statements are false

Directions summarised:

A:	True	True	second statement is **a correct explanation** of the first
B:	True	True	second statement is **NOT a correct explanation** of the first
C:	True	False	
D:	False	True	
E:	False	False	

Q9

■ *Statement 1*: Before starting the MUR the pharmacist should check that the patient has received information on the MUR and agreed to the process.
■ *Statement 2*: Patient consent must be obtained before commencing the MUR process.

Q10 This question is about the MUR on a patient that regularly takes co-codamol 8/500 effervescent tablets. The patient does not have difficulties swallowing tablets.

■ *Statement 1*: An action point on the MUR form could be to suggest that co-codamol is prescribed in tablet or capsule form.
■ *Statement 2*: Effervescent preparations have a high sodium content, which could be significant if the patient is taking regular doses.

Case studies

Level 1

Mr Daniels is 72 and suffers from osteoarthritis in both knees. He also has mild heart failure. He is overweight and does not smoke. Mr Daniels's PMR record is as follows:

- Paracetamol 500 mg tablets prn
- Co-codamol tablets 8/500 as directed
- Diclofenac 50 mg tds prn
- Furosemide 40 mg od
- Ramipril 5 mg od
- Simple linctus purchased from the supermarket.

From the PMR the pharmacist notices that he does not always order all of the medicine but always orders the paracetamol and co-codamol tablets. During the MUR he tells you that he has a troublesome cough and does not like taking so many tablets. He explains that he only takes either the paracetamol or the co-codamol depending on the severity of the pain.

- Using bullet points summarise the issues that need to be highlighted with this patient and their GP.

Level 2

Mary is 62 and has suffered from chronic obstructive pulmonary disease for many years. She used to smoke 20–30 cigarettes a day but has cut down on her smoking habit to 10 cigarettes a day. For the past 10 years she has taken:

- salbutamol inhaler 100 mcg 2 puffs prn
- ipratropium inhaler 2 puffs prn
- Beclazone inhaler 250 mcg 2 puffs bd
- Volmax tabs 8 mg 1 bd
- Slo-Phyllin caps 250 mg 2 bd.

On questioning during the MUR it appears that she has no problems taking all her medicines and according to the PMR record the medicines are ordered and supplied regularly.

Mary reports that she is reasonably well but has noticed that she seems to be increasingly breathless as the years go by. She also mentions that she has been getting palpitations for some time now and is concerned that there may be a problem with her heart.

- What areas would you need to explore before making your final action plan?

Level 3

Bill Jones has been working in community pharmacy for over 25 years. Bill's area manager is keen for him to offer an MUR service, and a suitable consultation room has been installed in the pharmacy. Bill is not very keen to offer this service as he does not feel he has the necessary clinical skills. However, after speaking to a colleague he is persuaded to attempt the Centre for Pharmacy Postgraduate Education (CPPE) online assessment and is successfully accredited.

In the first month after accreditation he conducts only three MURs and finds it very difficult to interest any of his regular customers in this service.

- What suggestions would you offer to Bill to increase the level of uptake of MURs in his pharmacy?

References

1   Department of Health. *A Vision for Pharmacy in the New NHS*. London: Department of Health, 2003. www.dh.gov.uk/en/Consultations/Closed consultations/DH_4068353 (accessed 7 September 2007).

2   Foulsham R, Siabi N, Nijjer S, Dhillon S. Ready steady, pause and take stock! Time to reflect on medicines use review. *Pharm J* 2006; **276**: 414.

3   Pharmaceutical Services Negotiating Committee. *Competency Framework for the Assessment of Pharmacists Providing the Medicines Use Review (MUR) and Prescription Intervention Service*. www.psnc.org.uk/uploaded_txt/Advanced_service_competency_framework.pdf (accessed 7 September 2007).

4   Pharmaceutical Services Negotiating Committee. *MURS: pharmacist accreditation options*. www.psnc.org.uk/index.php?type=more_news&id=1468 (accessed 7 September 2007).

5   Munro J, O'Caithan A, Knowles E, Nicholl J. Evaluation of NHS Direct 'referral' to community pharmacists. *Int J Pharm Pract* 2003; **11**: 1–9.

6   Pharmaceutical Services Negotiating Committee. *Application for Consent to Conduct an MUR Away from the Pharmacy (PREM2)*. www.psnc.org.uk/uploaded_txt/Form%20PREM2%20(PSNC).pdf (accessed 7 September 2007).

7   Pharmaceutical Services Negotiating Committee. *Community Pharmacy Contractual Framework, Advanced Service – Medicines Use Review & Prescription Intervention Service specification*. www.psnc.org.uk/uploaded_txt/Service%20Spec%20AS1%20-%20Medicines%20Use%20Review-Prescription%20Inter..pdf (accessed 7 September 2007).

8   Buisson J. How to make space for a consultation room in your community pharmacy. *Pharm J* 2005; **275**: 689–691.

9   Pharmaceutical Services Negotiating Committee. *Pharmacy Contractor Advance Services Requirements Premises Self-certification Form*. www.psnc.org.uk/uploaded_txt/Form%20PREM1%20_PSNC_.pdf (accessed 7 September 2007).

10   Pharmaceutical Services Negotiating Committee. Example of MUR

promotional material. www.psnc.org.uk/uploaded_txt/MUR%20Leaflet %20March%2006.pdf (accessed 7 September 2007).

11   Diabetes UK. *Balance* magazine. www.diabetes.org.uk/How_we_help/ Magazines_amp_publications/Balance/ (accessed 7 September 2007).

12   Pharmaceutical Services Negotiating Committee. LPC Briefing for GPs (Hampshire and Isle of Wight). www.psnc.org.uk/uploaded_txt/MUR %20LPC%20LMC%20Briefing%20Rev%20Oct06%20(2).pdf (accessed 7 September 2007).

13   NHS Employers. *Quality Outcomes Framework.* www.nhsemployers.org/ primary/primary-890.cfm (accessed 7 September 2007).

14   NHS. National Prescribing Centre. *Room for Review: a guide to medication review.* www.npc.co.uk/med_partnership/medication-review/room-for-review.html (accessed 7 September 2007).

15   Royal Pharmaceutical Society of Great Britain. Editorial (law and ethics bulletin). Interim guidance for pharmacist supervision and private consultation areas. *Pharm J* 2005; **275**: 756–758. www.pjonline.com/ Editorial/20051217/society/ethics.html#1 (accessed 11 September 2007).

16. Willcocks D. Medicines use reviews – uphill struggle. *Pharm J* 2005; **275**: 733.

17   Pharmaceutical Services Negotiating Committee. *Community Pharmacy Medicines Use Review & Prescription Intervention Service.* www.psnc.org. uk/uploaded_txt/Advanced%20Service%20Form.pdf (accessed 7 September 2007).

18   Alexander AM. MURs: how the picture is developing. *Pharm J* 2006; **276**: 44–46.

19   Blenkinsopp A, Gianpiero C, Bond C, Inch J. Medicines use reviews: the first year of a new community pharmacy service. *Pharm J* 2007; **278**: 218–220.

20   News feature. MURs: increasing quality and quantity. *Pharm J* 2007; **278**: 213. www.pjonline.com/Editorial/20070224/news/news_murs. html (accessed 11 September 2007).

Further information

- Useful companies to contact for compliance aids:
  - W&W Medsystems www.wwmed.co.uk
  - Dudley Hunt www.dudleyhunt.co.uk
  - Living Aids Ltd www.livingaidsonline.co.uk
  - PivoTell Ltd www.pivotell.co.uk

- Contacts for services for visually impaired (company that produce large print, Braille and other printed matter for the visually impaired)
  - A2i Transcription Services Ltd www.a2i.co.uk

6

Offering enhanced services

You create your opportunities by asking for them.

(Patty Hansen)

Checkpoint

Before reading on, think about the following questions to identify your own knowledge gaps in this area:

- What is a pharmaceutical needs assessment?
- What are the main barriers to the commissioning of pharmaceutical services?
- Name four enhanced services commonly commissioned by primary care trusts.
- What are some of the advantages of providing a minor ailments service?

Enhanced services form the third tier of the community pharmacy contract in England and Wales. These services are not part of the national contract; they are commissioned at a local level by primary care organisations (PCOs). A service specification for each enhanced service has been developed, using previous experience from locally negotiated services. In areas where it has been established that there is a need for a specific service, the individual contractors or local pharmaceutical committee (LPC) use the service specification as the basis for their negotiation with the PCO. An alternative approach is when the LPC, individual contractor or PCO develops their own bespoke service in response to identified local needs. The purpose of this chapter is to provide a practical guide to offering some of the more common enhanced services in the community and where to obtain further advice and support.

Commissioning of services

As enhanced services are only commissioned in response to the local needs of the population it is important that the pharmaceutical needs of the local population are assessed correctly. A full pharmaceutical needs assessment (PNA) is an important activity for all organisations planning local pharmaceutical services provision. For example, one of the key roles for pharmacy in public health is the assessment of the health and social needs of the population.[1] The National Primary and Care Trust Development Programme (NatPaCT) has developed a PNA toolkit that encourages the input of local community pharmacists into the planning process.[2] The importance of planning and supporting PNA is also emphasised in The National Pharmacy Association commissioning resource pack.[3] A study to identify and describe PNA activity in primary care trusts (PCTs) in England established that PNAs have been undertaken in most PCTs.[4] The study demonstrated that as a key stakeholder, local community pharmacists were engaged in the planning process in most PCTs.

The main barriers to the commissioning of pharmaceutical services, identified in a study of PCTs in England,[5] are access to funding, PCT capacity and reconfiguration and general practitioner (GP) support. Many pharmacists are unaware of the best way of sourcing funding and the PCT may have problems in the commissioning of services due to lack of staff and major changes in the way that funding is allocated. It has been demonstrated that services that depend on GP referral have low uptake rates.[6] It is important therefore that GPs are fully involved and informed of the commissioning process for this barrier to be overcome. At the time of writing the impact of the new contract on enhanced service commissioning levels has been modest.[7]

A list of enhanced services commissioned by PCTs and provided by community pharmacies is shown in Box 6.1. The highest rate of commissioning is for services for substance misuse and smoking-cessation services. This trend follows the national priority given to public health issues.

Costing of enhanced services

Initially, negotiations between the Pharmaceutical Services Negotiating Committee (PSNC), NHS Confederation and the Department of Health were aimed at producing benchmark prices for different enhanced services. The aim of this process was to publish a nationally agreed cost for the provision of each service. It was eventually agreed that a more practical approach would be to publish a pricing toolkit. The pricing toolkit has been developed by the PSNC. The toolkit is aimed at LPCs to use as a guide to ensure that specific cost elements are considered when costing a service. A set of elements to be allocated a cost for each enhanced service has been published by the PSNC.[8] The cost elements to be considered when offering an enhanced service are summarised in Table 6.1.

Box 6.1   Examples of possible enhanced services commissioned by PCTs and provided by community pharmacies

- Schools service
- Gluten-free foods
- Home-delivery service
- Anticoagulant monitoring
- Disease-specific medicines management
- Supplementary prescribing
- Screening service
- Language-access service
- Prescriber-support service
- Medication-review service
- Medicines-assessment and compliance support
- On-demand and specialist drugs
- Minor ailment scheme
- Out-of-hours
- Care-home service
- Patient group direction service
- Stop smoking
- Needle and syringe exchange
- Supervised administration
- Weight-management services
- Men's health check scheme

Table 6.1   Summary of the costs involved in setting up a new enhanced service

Cost element	Examples
Set-up/annual costs	Time to write business plan; risk-management assessments; time to establish a service level agreement (SLA)
Other costs	Equipment, insurance, travel costs, additional staff training
Service delivery	Labour costs, stock holding costs and consumables
Administration/review	Audit and management of review, meeting costs

The pricing toolkit designates the different sections of the template as always a cost, sometimes a cost or rarely a cost. For each service there are specific guidance notes that need to be considered when costing the service.

Example 6.1

If offering a service for the supervised administration of prescribed oral medicines such as methadone, it would be necessary to consider:

- an additional screened area for privacy
- the need for additional controlled drugs storage
- the need for specialist measuring equipment, for example a methadone pump to facilitate dispensing
- time involved in the administration process.

When costing services it is agreed that the cost of core pharmacy information technology (IT) requirements is covered by essential services funding. Any consultation room costs that are not used exclusively for an enhanced service may need to be taken from the provision of other services.

In Wales agreed prices have been published for certain services and there is an indication that in view of the low uptake of services in England and the limited budgets of PCTs, there is a need to be more specific about the prices of enhanced services. A possible solution is the publication of agreed prices for each element of an enhanced service but not a fixed benchmark price for the entire service.[9]

Practical guidance on delivering enhanced services

Support for care homes

The service description for this enhanced service states that the pharmacy will provide advice and support to the residents and staff within the care home, over and above the dispensing essential service.[10] The overall aim of this advisory service is to improve patient safety within the care home. The pharmacist will need to focus their attention on:

- ordering
- storage
- administration procedures
- disposal
- use of medicines, both prescribed and purchased.

Practical considerations

In order to be able to offer this service there are a number of practical considerations:

■ is the advisory support service to be provided by a different pharmacist from the pharmacist that supplies the home with regular medication? For example in some areas the pharmaceutical advice and support service has been provided by an individual pharmacist that has specialised in this area but does not supply the medication to the home. This option may be worth considering if there appears to be a local problem with the provision of this service
■ the more usual case is that the pharmacist offering the advisory support service is also the supplying pharmacist. The decision to become involved in this enhanced service may be linked to the decision to also supply the home with medication. The decision to offer a supply service will have many separate practical implications such as:
  – set-up costs
  – staff costs
  – staff training costs
  – space requirements
  – support for the supply function, such as the supply of interim medication and the delivery of medication.

The scope of this section is only concerned with the enhanced service of offering support and advice to the care home. The pharmacist will need to consider the following issues if they wish to become involved in offering support and advice to care homes:

■ accreditation with the local PCT to be able to offer this service. To be able to offer this service the pharmacist will need to be accredited by their local PCT. This will often involve the completion of a distance learning programme such as the Centre for Pharmacy Postgraduate Education (CPPE) care home training package,[11] and also attendance at locally arranged training events delivered by the PCT
■ time commitment and costs including the use of locum cover while off the premises visiting care homes and delivering training
■ information-management issues to comply with record-keeping requirements
■ liaison with PCT and inspecting pharmacists from the Commission for Social Care Inspection (CSCI)
■ provision of standard operating procedures for the support and advisory function.

The main areas of pharmacist involvement in service provision to care homes are outlined in Figure 6.1.

Pre-visit preparation for a new home

Before an initial visit, sufficient groundwork needs to be done to ensure that the first visit is as productive as possible. The initial work will include finding out the name of the main contact. This may be the owner of the home, a manager or a senior care worker who has been designated

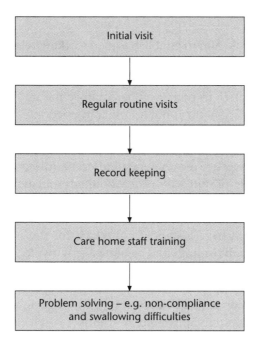

Figure 6.1 The main areas of pharmacist involvement in service provision to residential care homes.

specific responsibility for looking after the medication. If the care home offers nursing care, the visiting pharmacist will need to be in contact with the registered nurse in charge of the home. It is also useful to find out if there are any ongoing medication issues in the home or any major changes to the supply process. If there have been any specific problems with a resident's medication, the pharmacist may also need to liaise with local GPs or other community healthcare professionals.

A lot of time can be saved by the careful planning of a suitable time for the initial visit. This time will have to fit in with staff rotas to ensure that you see the most appropriate person and do not interrupt daily events such as mealtimes and medication rounds. It is useful to arrange a start time and a proposed finish time for the visit, so that the pharmacist can manage their time effectively and the care home staff are aware that the visit has a limited duration. To avoid any last-minute problems it is good practice to telephone the home shortly before the initial visit to confirm the appointment. In some cases a last-minute emergency that affects staffing arrangements will mean that the visit will have to be rearranged.

Initial visit

The first visit should aim to establish a good working relationship with the home and highlight any problem areas that require further attention. These areas can then be revisited on the regular routine visits. It is important at the outset to establish the advisory nature of the pharmacist visit and emphasise that it is not a formal inspection. The purpose of the initial visit is to provide an initial assessment of the systems for the management, storage and administration of medicines within the care home and to make appropriate recommendations. A useful starting point may be to ask the member of staff with responsibility for medication if they have any specific concerns. This may be a more open way of introducing the process rather than moving straight into the initial assessment process.

The PCT will have a standard checklist for the initial visit, which may have many subheadings and be quite a lengthy document. The pharmacist is more likely to gain useful information if the tone of the visit is supportive and helpful rather than judgemental. A conversational approach should be adopted when using this checklist, rather than asking a series of seemingly unrelated questions.

The areas of focus for the initial visit are:

- storage
- disposal
- documentation
- medicines profile record
- stock control systems
- medicine administration.

Storage

- Is the storage system suitable and secure and how are the keys accessed?
- Is the storage of medicines near the service users? If the medicine is stored some distance away this can lead to poor practices involving leaving medicines out in service users' rooms.
- Is there suitable storage for fridge items (with daily monitored and recorded maximum and minimum temperature)?
- Is there separate suitable storage of controlled drugs?
- What quantity of medication is stored? The amount of medication stored should relate to the monthly drug cycle. The pharmacist should check that any 'overflow medication' is not being stored in separate cupboards.
- Is the storage appropriate for the type of medication in the home? For example if the home uses predominantly blistered solid dose forms on racks there needs to be sufficient space to accommodate this system. If there is a large amount of liquid medication (for example large volumes of lactulose); is there adequate space?
- Is there separate storage of home remedies away from prescribed medication?

- Do service users that self-medicate have access to a lockable cupboard in their room?

Disposal

- Is there a system in place for the disposal of unwanted medication. For a residential home this currently means returning unwanted medication to a pharmacy. A nursing home would have to make arrangements with a specialist waste contractor.
- Are all returned unwanted medicines recorded?
- Is there any evidence of unsatisfactory waste-disposal methods such as flushing medication down the toilet?
- Is there a separate system in place for disposing of sharps and clinical waste?

Documentation

- Is it clear from the medicines administration record (MAR) sheet how the system of administration works?
- Are all doses accounted for, including the non-administration and a reason given?
- Do the dosage instructions on the MAR sheet match the instructions on the medication label?
- Is there any evidence of the MAR sheet being initialled retrospectively rather than at the time of administration? It would be expected that the MAR sheet would look like a working document with possible smudges and the irregular appearance of different initials. An MAR sheet that is too neat may need further investigation.
- Are the timings of the medicines appropriate?
- Do the quantities of medicine in storage match up to the expected quantity from the MAR sheet? It is useful to spot check certain items to check that there are no discrepancies that cannot be explained.

Medicines profile record

Each service user should have a medicines profile that records all medicines being taken and the start and finish date. The medicines pro-file record should also record details of the prescriber and a clear state-ment of any drug allergies. The pharmacist should check medicines profile cards against MAR sheets to ensure that the information correlates and that the medicines profile gives suitable additional information.

Stock control systems

Strictly speaking, the term stock is misleading as all medication in a care home is prescribed and is the property of the individual. On the initial visit the pharmacist should check that all medicines coming into the home are signed for and a record is made of all medicines administered, discontinued or returned as unwanted. In many cases this system is incorporated into the MAR sheet, but in some homes there are separate stock record cards.

Medicine administration

- What type of monitored dose system is being used? In smaller homes a monitored dosage system is not always in place. The pharmacist should check that the system in place is suitable for the type and size of home.
- What procedures are in place to identify the service user before giving medicine?
- Is there any evidence of 'borrowing' medication from one service user to be given to another service user?
- What systems are in place to assess service users for self-medication?
- Are there any issues surrounding service users who have swallowing difficulties? The practice of crushing solid dose forms and the covert administration of medicines may be an issue, and this is discussed later in this chapter.

Regular routine visits

As part of the service specification, routine follow-up visits should be undertaken at least every 6 months. The aim of the regular visits is to work on the areas that have been identified in the initial visit as needing attention. Changes to specific areas should be recorded and in some cases the home may need reminding of areas that still require attention. Once the regular systems in place are satisfactory, the follow-up visits can be used to keep a check that standards are being maintained. This should take less time as the visits progress and the pharmacist will have more time to spend on such issues as:

- individual service users' medication. This may take the form of a simple medication review for suitable service users who wish to speak to a pharmacist about their medication. This review will need to be done in the presence of a member of staff and adequate time should be allowed for a meaningful interaction
- assisting staff with protocols and procedures that relate to medication usage
- the discussion of the use of home remedies and healthy lifestyle issues
- systematically reviewing all medication for each service user from the MAR sheets.

Pharmacist record keeping

Individual PCTs have their own service outline and specific recording documentation for pharmacist visits. The pharmacy must have in place a written agreement with the care home to provide this service. This agreement usually relates to a financial year and has the provision for termination of the contract on either side by providing an agreed period of notice. A copy of the agreement to provide this support and advisory service is lodged with the PCT. For the purposes of ongoing service delivery and audit a full record of all advice given to the home on each visit must be recorded. The usual procedure would be for a pharmacist to document each visit with the date, time and name of the responsible person in charge at the time of the visit. Any issues discussed would be detailed and both the pharmacist and the representative from the home would sign the documentation. A copy of the visit notes would be sent to the PCT and a further copy sent to the manager of the home for information. The original copy would be retained by the pharmacist and filed securely. On future visits, reference should be made to previous action plans to ensure satisfactory progress towards desired outcomes. For clinical governance it is vital that the pharmacist can refer back to previous visits and any areas that have been found to be deficient. It is useful to refer back to the initial visit document and make a note of the date and subsequent significant improvements, in order to close the loop.

Care home staff training

One of the aims and intended service outcomes of this advisory service is to provide training to help improve the skills of the care home staff. This type of training can be informal and is often incorporated into the regular visit to the home. In practice, on-the-job training in a care home can be difficult to achieve as the care worker is often very busy. A more practical alternative is for the pharmacist to provide a more formal and structured training session. This type of training is more popular as it provides the home with certified evidence of recognised staff training in the area of medicines administration. Training at this level is over and above the service specification, and has cost implications in terms of pharmacist time, venue hire and training materials; therefore a charge would be levied for each attendee. There may be local opportunities for pharmacists to become involved in offering this type of external training service to care homes.

Resolving common problems

Swallowing difficulties

A common problem raised by care workers is the issue of facilitating service users' swallowing of solid-dose forms. The visiting pharmacist can sometimes become involved in providing advice in this area.

The widespread practice of crushing tablets and opening capsules is of particular concern.[12] There is increasing evidence that crushing tablets or capsules which are enteric coated or have slow-release properties may be harmful to the patient. There is also a legal issue, as by crushing a solid-dose form the product is then being administered outside its product licence.

If the pharmacist is presented with a swallowing difficulty issue, the use of alternative formulations should be explored as fully as possible, including the use of a specials manufacturer. If an alternative formulation is not available and crushing the dose form appears to be the only option, the next stage is to check if the medicine can be safely crushed or opened. For example, it would be inappropriate for hormonal, cytotoxic or steroidal drugs to be crushed, as the powder may go into the air and present a risk to the person administering the dose.

The crushing of tablets is seen as a last resort and if it is decided to go ahead with this course of action, permission must be obtained from the prescriber and patient or their representative. It should be made clear to the prescriber that the crushed medicine is being administered in an unlicensed form and a full record made in the patient's care plan.

Conflicts of interest

Occasionally problems may arise due to the home not heeding the advice of the pharmacist. If the supplying and advising pharmacist is the same person this can sometimes cause relationship difficulties with the home. It should be emphasised that the supply and advisory role are two separate functions, even though the home may believe that there is a commercial interest for the pharmacist in retaining the home business. If problems of non-compliance with specific local procedures arise and the problems cannot be resolved after clear reminders, it is important that the problem is made transparent. In some cases it is necessary to report the home to the inspecting authority for further investigation. This is vital if the care of service users is compromised. The pharmacist must act within their professional code of ethics to ensure that the best interests of the service user are always considered

Quality indicators for the service

The suggested quality indicators for the service are:

- any routine visits by a care home inspection organisation do not highlight any major shortfalls in the systems of medicines management
- the pharmacy has an annual review of the standard operating procedures and referral pathways for this service

- pharmacy staff involved in this service can demonstrate that they have undertaken relevant continuing professional development (CPD)
- the pharmacy participates in any PCO audit of the service or any initiative involving the assessment of service user experience.

Smoking-cessation services

Background

In addition to the obvious human costs of increased premature death and morbidity, there are massive financial costs associated with smoking. It is estimated that smoking costs the NHS an estimated £1.5 billion every year.[13] To make a significant impact on smoking-related mortality and morbidity it is important to concentrate on smoking cessation rather than on policies to prevent people taking up smoking. There is little evidence that prevention policies work.[14] Smoking is increasingly concentrated in poorer socio-economic groups and consequently makes a significant contribution to health inequalities. The white paper, *Smoking Kills*,[15] has the ambitious target of a 1.5 million reduction in adult smokers by the year 2010. For the first time in the history of the NHS, resources are being invested in new smoking-cessation services to help smokers who want to give up. The introduction of the NHS Stop Smoking service, which combines psychological support with provision of smoking cessation products, is the first time this type of service has been introduced. The results are encouraging, as the latest figures show that in one year over half a million people who had contact with the service had set a quit date.[16] Out of this half a million people, over half had stopped smoking after the quit date. Pharmacies are recognised as being well placed to offer a smoking-cessation service as they are readily accessed by the public and have a resident healthcare professional.

The 'stop smoking' service commissioned by PCTs and provided by community pharmacies is one of the most popular enhanced services being provided.[17] Specific details of delivering the service vary according to locally agreed guidelines. For example the provision of nicotine-replacement therapy (NRT) can be made either by patient group directions (PGD) or by supplementary prescribing. The following practical guidelines assume that the NRT is provided by means of a PGD.

Aims of the service

One of the aims and intended service outcomes as outlined in the 'stop smoking' service specification is to improve access to and choice of stop smoking services.[18] This includes access to both pharmacological and non-pharmacological stop smoking aids. Smoking-cessation services are classified as:

- brief interventions which are defined as opportunistic advice from a healthcare professional delivered during a routine consultation
- intermediate interventions which are defined as one-to-one, face-to-face behavioural support over a 4-week period, delivered by someone trained in smoking cessation
- specialist support defined as the provision of behavioural support and advice delivered in a clinic or group run by a stop smoking specialist.

Pharmacists are involved routinely in brief interventions as part of the essential service promoting healthy lifestyles. There are many occasions when interacting with patients that it becomes apparent that smoking-cessation advice would be appropriate.

The enhanced service 'stop smoking' would be classed as an intermediate intervention and the details of the service would be specified by the PCT. In general terms this involves a pharmacist undergoing smoking-cessation training and offering a one-to-one client support service over a 4-week period. The provision of NRT products as part of a PGD means that patients who are normally exempt from prescription charges do not have to pay for this service.

Staff training

To be able to offer this service the pharmacist is required to attend smoking-cessation training sessions. The training sessions are normally provided by the smoking-cessation lead for the local PCT and include training evenings and distance learning materials. The management and monitoring of a PGD protocol for NRT is jointly approved by a multidisciplinary group including doctor, pharmacist and other healthcare professionals involved in delivering the service. Each individual pharmacist needs to be authorised to supply NRT under the PGD and receives written authorisation from the PCT. The training includes information on how to offer client support in the smoking-cessation process, information on the NRT products and administration details for using the PGD.

General principles of NRT

NRT delivers nicotine in a clean form and helps smokers to overcome withdrawal symptoms such as irritability and craving while avoiding the many harmful chemicals in tobacco and the carbon monoxide that cause serious damage. There are many different forms of NRT available including patches, gum, sublingual tablets, lozenges, inhalators and nasal spray. It is a useful exercise to refer to the manufacturer's literature for each product to become familiar with the dosing and practical issues associated with each dosage form.

The choice of product will depend on a number of factors including:

- smoking habits
- behavioural dependence
- patient preference
- previous quitting experience
- convenience of use.

Patches continue to be a popular option as they can be applied easily and compliance is not usually an issue. The disadvantage is that they do not offer any support for the smoker that is behaviourally dependent. An oral product would be more suitable for a behaviourally dependent smoker. The patch can also induce a mild skin reaction. The recommended length of treatment is 3 months and it is important that the patient does not smoke at all while using NRT.

If NRT gum is selected, the client should be advised not to eat or drink for 15 minutes before using or while chewing. Drinks such as orange juice or coffee should also be avoided around the same time, as they can reduce the effectiveness of the product. The correct chewing technique to obtain sufficient blood nicotine levels is to chew the gum slowly until the taste becomes strong and then place ('park') the gum between the cheek and the gum so allowing absorption through the buccal membrane. The repeated process of chewing and parking should be continued for about 30 minutes. Side-effects such as a sore mouth or throat are often transient and the client should be aware that there are pH changes in the mouth after stopping smoking, which may be the cause of the irritation.

The inhalator device is more suitable for highly behaviour-dependent smokers who will miss the hand-to-mouth action. Sublingual tablets are more suitable for smokers with an irregular smoking pattern and smokers who want to use a more discreet NRT product. Lozenges are also suitable for smokers with an irregular smoking pattern who smoke fewer than 20 cigarettes a day. If the smoker is highly dependent and needs rapid relief from cravings, the use of a nasal spray may be more appropriate.

Initial assessment

As part of the service outline the pharmacist is required to use a private consultation room and comply with national and local guidelines. The service is accessed by one of three routes:

- pharmacy referral as a result of the promotion of healthy lifestyles (public health) or signposting essential services
- direct referral by the individual
- referral by another health or social care worker.

The pharmacist would need to confirm the eligibility of the person to access the service, based on local guidelines. A wide range of advertising material is available from the PCT smoking-cessation lead to inform interested clients of the availability of this service.

Table 6.2 Summary of the stages involved in stopping smoking (Prochaska and DiClemente[19])

Stage	Support	Client response
Precontemplation stage	No action necessary	The client has no interest in changing behaviour and still sees personal advantages in continuing to smoke
Preparation stage	Suggest best ways to stop and offer encouragement	There are some thoughts about changing and some of the dangers of smoking are acknowledged. The client is not quite ready as they still have reasons for continuing the smoking habit
Action stage		There is the implementation of lifestyle changes and the client has stopped smoking
Maintenance stage	Keep client motivated and continue support programme	The client believes that stopping is a possibility and has made a definite plan to stop. They can see that stopping could bring personal benefit
Relapse	Ensure that client is aware that support is available when they are ready to attempt to quit again	The client has started smoking again and left the 'stop smoking' programme. It is important that the client is advised about coping strategies to come out of this stage
Permanent quit of smoking	No further action necessary	

The initial assessment should include an assessment of the person's readiness to make a quit attempt and also their willingness to use appropriate treatments.

Areas for discussion that can be included in the first meeting are:

- identification of reasons for smoking and why the smoker wishes to quit smoking
- talking through a typical day or week and when smoking takes place and why smoking takes place at these times
- discussion of high-risk situations when the smoker is more likely to smoke and asking the smoker to identify what they could do instead of smoking.

Work done by Prochaska and DiClemente resulted in a 'cycle of change' model which suggests that stopping smoking is not a single event but rather a process in which the smoker goes through a series of stages (Table 6.2).[19]

During the initial meeting it is important to explore the client's motivation for stopping smoking. If there appears to be a genuine motivation to stop smoking the pharmacist can provide a lot of positive support and encouragement (Box 6.2).

Box 6.2   Useful hints and tips for the first few days of quitting

---

- Plan a quit date that is relatively stress free and when support is available. Make a note of the quit date and stick to this date.
- Concentrate on the benefits of not smoking and ask friends and family for support.
- Avoid situations where you usually smoke.
- Give the project of stopping smoking first priority.
- Never have just one cigarette as this brings you back to the beginning.
- See yourself as a non-smoker.
- Take one day at a time.
- Think in advance about strategies for coping with stress, temptation, cravings and weight gain.

During the initial session a monitoring form will be filled in with the client's details. This form should include details of how many cigarettes a day the client smokes, smoking history and an indication of previous quit attempts. The quit attempt history should include a record of any NRT products used, how long they stopped smoking for and how useful they found particular products.

The initial session should also include:

- a general explanation of NRT
- the selection of a suitable product for the client
- a discussion of the practical aspects of using NRT and giving up
- setting a specific quit date
- provision of useful support materials such as a 'Days stopped smoking' chart.

The initial supply of NRT should be made 2 weeks from the target quit date. If the client continues to stop smoking then further supplies are given with the offer of weekly support. The support may be by telephone if appropriate. An appointment should be made for 2 weeks after the quit date. Each consultation or contact is documented on the client record card.

Follow-up consultations

Two weeks after the quit date the client is invited to discuss openly how the quit is progressing and any problems identified. If necessary the NRT may be changed and further advice given on how to persist when cravings are present. The third week after the quit date should include a positive recognition of the successful quit attempt. The aim at this stage is to motivate the client and emphasise any positive changes.

The 4-week follow-up should include a self-reported smoking status and this should be validated by a carbon monoxide breath test. This is a motivational device that provides some quantitative measurement, as the level of carbon monoxide in the lungs decreases when the smoker stops smoking. If the client is successful at stopping smoking at this stage they should be issued with another 4 weeks of NRT. If the smoker is unsuccessful in stopping smoking at 4 weeks then they should discontinue treatment and a fresh start made when they are ready to quit smoking again. It is normally another 6 months before NHS funding is provided for another attempt.

If the smoker has successfully stopped at 8 weeks then another 2–4 weeks' supply can be given. If at 10–12 weeks the smoker has still been successful, then treatment should be gradually withdrawn at this point.

Quality indicators

Suggested quality indicators for this service include:

- provision of appropriate health-promotion material provided by the pharmacy
- annual review of standard operating procedures for this service and the referral pathways

- demonstration of relevant CPD by pharmacists and staff involved in the delivery of this service
- comparison of the 4-week quit rate with the PCT target
- participation in an annual audit of service and assessment of service user experience by the PCO.

Minor ailments service

There is a significant emphasis on encouraging people to take more responsibility for looking after their health. This is demonstrated by the introduction of NHS Direct, provision of walk-in centres and the reclassification of some prescription only medicines (POMs) to pharmacy medicine (P) status. The self-care agenda is further underlined in the new contractual framework with the emphasis on self-care and the provision for minor ailments schemes as an enhanced service.

A minor ailments service is the supply of medicines by the NHS through community pharmacies from a limited formulary. The service is free of charge to patients who are exempt from prescription charges. This removes the payment barrier and encourages patients to access pharmacies and relieve the pressure on GPs for the treatment of minor ailments. It is estimated that between 20% and 40% of GP time is spent on minor ailments and some research shows that one in three GP consultations is for a minor illness.[20]

The aim of this enhanced service is to improve access and choice for people with minor ailments. The scheme is based on the provision of advice and, where appropriate, medicines and dressings, which would otherwise have been obtained on a prescription from a GP. The service depends on a referral system from local medical practices or other primary care providers and aims to reduce medical practice workload relating to minor ailments.

Service outline

The service outline covers the following areas:

- there should be a sufficient level of privacy that meets locally agreed criteria. Local arrangements will vary but in many cases this will involve talking to the patient at the medicines counter area with the option for using a consultation room when necessary
- pharmacists and staff involved in the service are appropriately trained. This may involve distance learning or bespoke training with the PCT to ensure that pharmacy staff are clear about how the service will operate
- pharmacists and staff involved in the service are aware of local protocols and operate within the agreed framework. The protocol will include all areas of the service including the means of referral to the scheme, outline

treatment pathways for the list of conditions included, record-keeping requirements and the operation of a triage system which includes referral to other health and social care professionals where appropriate
- the pharmacy maintains records of the service to ensure ongoing service delivery and audit. The PCO will specify what records are to be maintained and how this information is collected and used
- there is a local minor ailments formulary. Within previously commissioned schemes a number of conditions have been included (Box 6.3). For each condition there is a recommended course of action and agreed product recommendation
- the PCO has agreed which groups of people are eligible to receive treatment under the scheme and how the scheme is accessed. Access to the scheme may be by one of three methods:
  - local access where any patient registered with a local GP practice that is participating in the scheme can present in the pharmacy
  - a voucher scheme where the patient needs a voucher to access the scheme
  - referral by another healthcare team member.

Box 6.3 Examples of minor ailments that have been commonly included within previously commissioned local schemes

---

- Back ache, sprains and strains
- Colds
- Conjunctivitis
- Constipation
- Coughs
- Diarrhoea
- Earache
- Haemorrhoids
- Hayfever
- Head lice
- Headache and fever
- Heartburn and indigestion
- Insect bites and stings
- Mild eczema and dermatitis
- Minor fungal infections of the skin
- Mouth ulcers
- Nappy rash
- Sore throat
- Teething
- Threadworm
- Thrush

To participate in the scheme, the pharmacy agrees to provide advice on the management of the specific minor ailments or to provide advice and a medicine from the local formulary. In some cases it is necessary to provide advice on the management of the ailment and refer the patient to an appropriate healthcare professional. The pharmacy also agrees to maintain a record of the consultation and any medicine that has been supplied. The scheme has a standard form that can be used for each consultation and a system of checking a person's eligibility for access to the service and the payment of NHS charges where applicable.

The PCO will be responsible for supporting and administering the service locally. This will include the provision of supporting materials for the public and also information relevant to pharmacy staff such as signposting information.

Setting up a service

To be able to set up this service pharmacists will need to be proactive and may have to convince the local PCT of the value of minor ailments schemes. This will mean liaising with pharmacy development groups and LPCs to make a case for releasing finance for this enhanced service. The National Pharmacy Association has a toolkit for setting up a minor ailments scheme.[21] Setting up a new service will involve a substantial amount of preliminary work before the scheme can be implemented. The first stage is to research the PCT's stated aims for the healthcare of its population and carry out a needs assessment to see how the scheme would fit into any existing local provision. For example it will be necessary to consider existing minor ailments clinics in GP surgeries and be able to promote the benefit of improved access through pharmacies. Once this research has been completed a strategy for development of the service will need to be drafted. A summary of the main areas to be agreed on in order to implement a minor ailments scheme is outlined in Figure 6.2.

Suggested quality indicators

Possible quality indicators for a minor ailments service include:

- the use and uptake of PCO promotional material
- annual review of standard operating procedures and the referral pathways for the scheme
- demonstration of relevant CPD by staff involved in this service
- participation in annual PCO audit of service provision including satisfaction surveys of service users.

Studies have shown that people who have accessed a minor ailments service have found it to be effective in providing rapid and convenient

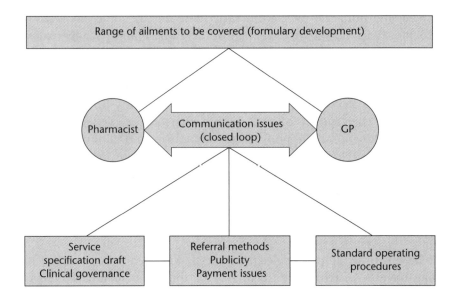

Figure 6.2 Summary of the main areas for consideration when setting up a minor ailments scheme.

access to advice and treatment.[22] There is increasing evidence of the benefits of providing this innovative enhanced service.

Needle and syringe exchange

Background

A needle and syringe exchange scheme is the provision of a service where injecting drug users can obtain sterile injecting equipment, free of charge, in exchange for their used ones. Provision of this service has always been a controversial issue particularly in the late 1980s when the scheme was launched in the UK. At the time of the introduction of the scheme the government appeared to be sending out mixed messages as there was a 'Just say no' anti-heroin campaign at the time. The 1980s also brought increasing evidence that the sharing of syringes resulted in large increases in HIV infection among injecting drug users. The principle of harm reduction began to emerge as part of an overall strategy to respond to the potential rise in HIV infection. It was recognised that HIV and AIDS presented a greater threat to the individual and public health than drug misuse.

The World Health Organization states that there is compelling evidence that increasing the availability of and utilisation of sterile injecting equipment by intravenous drug users reduces HIV infection substantially.[23] Studies show a lower HIV prevalence rate among syringe exchange clients.[24] However, exchange schemes have had little impact on high-risk sexual risk behaviour, which for intravenous drug misusers may be the main route of transmission of HIV.

Needle and syringe exchange schemes offered by pharmacies are successful due to the ease of accessibility and the presence of a healthcare professional who can be seen without appointment. A national survey of community pharmacists' attitudes and their involvement in service-specific training, concluded that pharmacists were positive about their role in HIV prevention and the provision of clean injecting equipment to injecting drug users.[25] The positive attitude was more evident among pharmacists who were already offering the service. This study also demonstrated that only a minority of pharmacists had participated in any training on drug misuse and HIV prevention.

A study to determine if pharmacy customers are deterred from using a pharmacy that offers services to drug misusers demonstrated that generally pharmacy customers were supportive of needle and syringe exchange schemes, provided there was adequate privacy in the pharmacy.[26] The issue of shoplifting and violence should not deter the pharmacist from offering this service. A clear zero tolerance of any threatening or abusive conduct should be made clear to the client at the outset of offering the service. The successful operation of this service is all about mutual respect and clear guidelines of acceptable behaviour.

Practical issues for the pharmacist

The Royal Pharmaceutical Society of Great Britain (RPSGB) *Medicines, Ethics and Practice* guide (MEP) provides information on practice guidance documents.[27] 'Best practice guidance for commissioners and providers of pharmaceutical services for drug users' includes service principles for the provision of a pharmacy needle exchange scheme.

The practical issues to consider when offering this service are the physical environment, available equipment, disposal of equipment and staff training.

The part of the pharmacy used for the provision of an exchange service must provide a sufficient level of privacy and safety. Depending on the number of service users it may be necessary to have a clearly defined area that is situated away from the main prescription reception and medicine counter area. If the service only involves a few clients a month then it would be sufficient to have a sharps bin under a counter out of view and a supply of clean exchange equipment in a secure and easily accessible drawer. The position of all equipment and disposal bins needs to be well out of public reach. The pharmacy should display a logo such as the established double arrow logo (Figure 6.3) that is recognised by service users, or an equivalent local logo that indicates participation in the service. The pharmacy is not required to advertise the service in their practice leaflet.

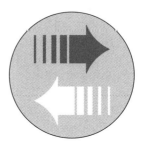

Figure 6.3   National logo for pharmacy needle exchange scheme.

The smooth operating of the service depends on having a clear protocol for the exchange process. The pharmacy may have a system of only exchanging during quiet periods to reduce any disruption to the normal flow of work. This policy will depend on the size of pharmacy and if there is a separate designated area for the exchange to take place. It should only be the pharmacist or suitably trained member of staff who is involved with the service user.

The first stage is to ask the client if they have anything to return. If the client has nothing to return they should be asked how they have disposed of their old equipment and strong advice given on making returns of used equipment in the future. In some cases the service user may have disposed of the equipment in a legitimate way through another pharmacy or used another sharps container. However, if the disposal has been through an unacceptable means such as public litter bin or household waste, the service user needs reminding of the specific returns policy for the system to operate successfully. The pharmacist may wish to negotiate with the local scheme manager if an individual returns policy can be adopted by the pharmacy. The main practical issue is providing a consistent message to service users in the event on non-returned equipment. When the client produces their used equipment, which should be in the small sharps bin, the pharmacist or staff member should not handle the item. The used complete pack should be placed directly in the pharmacy sharps container that is designated specifically for this purpose. For this system to operate smoothly, the position of the pharmacy sharps bin needs careful consideration. Most systems involve issuing all clients with a unique reference number either on a card or a key ring. The number is then quoted at the time of each exchange so that the pharmacist can record details of all exchanges that take place. This information will be required for payment and audit purposes. New clients should be registered using a client registration form. To preserve anonymity, the information collected should not extend further than details such as initials, age, sex, postcode and the substances that are being injected. This confidential information is useful for monitoring drug misuse in a locality.

As part of the service outline the pharmacy contractor should ensure that staff are aware of the risk associated with handling returned used equipment and the correct procedures to minimise risk. A needle-stick injury procedure should be in place and all staff involved in this service should be offered immunisation for hepatitis B. The receipt of unprotected dirty needles is unusual, and in the unlikely event of a needlestick injury bleeding should be encouraged and the injured site washed thoroughly with hot running water. The GP or hospital emergency department should be contacted and a record of the accident made.

The new equipment offered to the service user will depend on the local scheme that is being operated. Some schemes offer pre-packed small sharps containers containing syringes, needles, swabs, condoms and an information leaflet. In some cases the scheme protocol may allow the client to select equipment items from a limited range. This 'pick and mix' system is thought to be more economical but has the disadvantage of being more time consuming as more interaction is required. After the exchange process has taken place and the necessary records made there should be an opportunity for the client to ask any health-related questions. One of the intended service outcomes is to reinforce harm-reduction messages. This would include advice on safe sex and the risks associated with overdose, poly-drug and alcohol use. An integral part of the service is to help the service user to access other health and social care providers and act as a gateway to other services, for example services such as key working, specialist prescribing, hepatitis B immunisation, hepatitis and HIV screening and primary care services.

The PCO will provide all the exchange packs and the associated materials and will commission a clinical waste-disposal service to regularly service the pharmacy. The frequency of the waste collection should be agreed according to the level of service use. It is unacceptable to allow the build-up of clinical waste on pharmacy premises.

Types of syringes and needles
The most popular disposable plastic syringe is the U100 0.5 ml or 1 ml insulin syringe with a fine needle suitable for intravenous use. The 0.5 ml syringe is more suited to drug misusers who inject subcutaneously as the needles are small. This type of syringe has the needle fixed to the syringe so it would be useful to offer a means of clipping the needle such as a BD needle-clipping device. This will ensure safer disposal of the syringe. Larger syringes such as 2 ml, 5 ml or 10 ml are more suited to users who are injecting large volumes. These syringes have a luer mount and can take different sizes of needle. Needles are often identified by colour and length. The colour of the mount of the needle indicates the gauge or diameter of the needle. The most popular needle sizes are shown in Table 6.3.

Table 6.3   Summary of the most popular needle sizes used in needle-exchange schemes

Colour	Gauge (diameter in mm)	Length (mm)
Orange	25G (0.5)	16, 25
Blue	23G (0.6)	25, 30
Green	21G (0.8)	25, 40, 50

The longer needle sizes need a thicker diameter or gauge for strength.

In terms of reducing the amount of damage to the body, the finest needle possible should be selected. A short fine needle is suitable for injecting into good veins but a longer and thicker needle is needed if the veins are more difficult to locate. Drug misusers injecting steroids or without good veins present will inject intramuscularly into the buttock or thigh and will tend to use a longer blue or green needle. The smaller-gauge orange needle is likely to snap off in this type of injection. In some cases there is the practice of drawing up the solution from the ampoule with a large-gauge needle then swapping to a smaller-gauge needle for the injection. Needles with integral filters are available, which are useful for filtering street drugs. This type of needle needs to be changed to a standard needle before the injection. The prohibitive high cost of this type of needle reduces their widespread use in exchange schemes. Clients can often complain about the quality of the equipment provided and sometimes believe it is of an inferior quality. The main complaints can be that the barrel of the syringe is stiff or the needles are blunt. Tact and diplomacy are needed to communicate the message that the equipment is designed for high-quality pharmaceuticals and not heavily cut 'street drugs'.

Injecting drug misusers may develop a number of health problems such as skin infections, and sometimes approach the pharmacist for practical advice. This is a specialised area and it may be appropriate to undertake some CPD in this area if offering this service. Suggested reading on this subject can be found at the end of this chapter.

Suggested quality indicators

Suggested quality indicators include:

- meeting the locally agreed targets for return rates of used equipment
- availability of suitable health-promotion material and the promotion of its uptake
- appropriate CPD for pharmacists and the team involved in delivering the service
- participation in an annual PCO audit and assessment of service user experience
- annual review of the standard operating procedures and the referral pathways for the service.

Supervised administration (consumption of prescribed medicines)

Background

This service involves the pharmacist in supervision of the consumption of prescribed medication at the point of dispensing, to ensure that the dose has been administered to the patient. The pharmacy will also provide advice and support to the patient, including referral to primary care or specialist centres where appropriate. The most common example of this type of service is the supervised administration of methadone. This service specification can also be applied to medicines used for the management of mental health conditions and tuberculosis.

The supervision of methadone consumption reduces the amount of illicit methadone leaking on to the streets.[28] Other advantages of the scheme include a reduction in the risks of loss or theft of the drug. There is also a reduction in bingeing, injecting and overdose cases. As the trust between doctors and patients is enhanced and the treatment programme progresses, the patient can gradually be allowed to take a one-day supply home. The Advisory Council on the Misuse of Drugs recommends that all opiate addicts being newly treated with methadone should have to take their methadone under daily supervision for at least 6 months.[29] In many cases the supervision period is much less than this and the client is rewarded with 'take home' doses if there is good compliance with the supervised regimen. In practice, new treatment of opiate dependence is subject to supervised consumption for a period of 3 months. This provides a clear routine and structure for the client and helps the client to distance themselves from erratic and risky behaviour. Pharmacists considering becoming involved in this service can access a number of useful references that describe the rationale and the practical issues involved in offering this service.[30]

Service outline

The issue of privacy and safety is of particular concern when offering this service. The most convenient arrangement is a separate hatch with a buzzer that opens on to the dispensing area. The hatch can only be opened from the inside and privacy is offered to the client by a booth or kiosk surrounding the area. This ensures that service users do not interrupt the prescription reception area. The methadone should be provided in a suitable receptacle such as a plastic medicine tumbler. Water should be provided after the administration to ensure that the dose has been swallowed. This reduces the risk of doses being held in the mouth and being regurgitated later. If the client does not want a drink the pharmacist should ascertain that the dose has been taken by asking the client to verbally confirm that the dose has been taken. A three-way agreement is set up between the prescriber, pharmacist and service user. The agreement covers all areas of how the service will operate, including specified times that the service is available and norms of acceptable behaviour for the service to operate. There should be a clear agreement about the action to be taken if there is non-compliance by the client. When drawing up the agreement with a new client it is useful to arrange a mutually convenient time for the supervised administration, so that busy dispensing periods are avoided. In many cases the agreement is a four-way contract that also involves the client's key worker who is often the first point of contact if problems arise.

To avoid any delay to the client, all instalments should be made up in advance and the quantities double checked and signed for audit purposes. A decision will need to be made on the purchase of a metered-dose methadone pump to ease the dispensing process. All prepared methadone instalments should remain in the locked controlled drugs (CD) cabinet until the time of dispensing. Under no circumstances should the client's methadone be poured directly from a stock bottle directly into a medicine tumbler. The pharmacy must not deviate from the instruction given on the prescription in terms of the type of methadone supplied. For example, sugar-free and colour-free products have a greater potential for abuse than syrup-based and coloured products. Sugar- and colour-free products must not be dispensed unless specifically prescribed. Most supervised schemes allow supplies to be taken home for Sundays and Bank Holidays. The pharmacist must ensure that they operate within the locally agreed protocol and have undertaken any additional training recommended by the PCO.

Methadone for instalment dispensing is prescribed on a blue FP10 MDA 'drugs misuse instalment prescription' form and the pharmacist maintains a record of all instalments supplied on the form. There is also a locally produced form for the supervised scheme, to record all supervised administration and this also requires a signature from the pharmacist and the client. All of these records are in addition to the legal record required in the CD register. The RPSGB issues clear guidance about instalment dispensing. For example, if an instalment prescription covers more than one day and is not collected on the specified day, the total amount prescribed less the amount prescribed for the day(s) missed may be supplied. However, as part of the initial contract with the client it is important to set up specific ground rules. The agreed ground rules should include details of the consequences of a missed dose and at what point the key worker or prescriber is informed of a missed dose.

Sometimes the client requests to purchase injecting equipment and it may be that the pharmacy does not offer a needle- and syringe-exchange service. The current guidance is that only in exceptional circumstances should pharmacists supply clean injecting equipment for drug misusers. The client must always be advised of availability of disposal facilities at the pharmacy and be encouraged to dispose of used syringes and needles safely. It is important that all staff involved in the delivery of this service are trained to treat service users with courtesy and respect.

A pharmacist who is new to providing a supervised methadone service should be aware of some of the potentially difficult requests or situations that may arise. This client group can be unreliable in adhering to agreed guidelines and may present seemingly plausible requests in order to obtain their supply of methadone. The pharmacist must ensure that they are adequately prepared to offer this service and undertake appropriate CPD. The CPPE distance learning materials on drug use and misuse and a series of practical case studies with suggested answers provide a useful insight into offering this service.[31,32]

Other supervised schemes

The supervision of the consumption of medicines used in the treatment of people with mental illness has a number of advantages:

- a regular pattern of attendance and consumption of the prescribed medication can help to reduce chaotic and risky behaviour patterns in this patient group
- regular contact with the pharmacist can help to reduce social isolation that is a feature of mental illness
- the pharmacist and pharmacy team are well placed to detect any deterioration of a person's mental state and can inform other members of the healthcare team that further support is needed

Directly Observed Therapy Schemes (DOTSs) have been used in many countries to improve full compliance with medication treatment regimens for tuberculosis. This condition is an increasing problem especially amongst socially disadvantaged groups such as the homeless. Effective treatment and the prevention of acquired drug resistance depend on full compliance with the prescribed regimen. There is some evidence that supervised treatment compared to self-treatment results in a higher incidence of treatment-completion rates.[33]

Suggested quality indicators

There are similar suggested quality indicators for this service as for the needle- and syringe-exchange scheme. The quality indicators are based on the provision of suitable health-promotion material, appropriate CPD for participating pharmacists, review of standard operating procedures and compliance with PCO audit.

Implications for practice

Activity 1

Find out from your local PCT what local pharmaceutical needs and objectives have been identified.

- How were these pharmaceutical needs identified?
- What progress has been made towards achieving the objectives?

Activity 2

Discuss with a colleague their experiences of providing an enhanced service.

- How did they work out the costs involved in providing the service?
- What are the advantages and disadvantages of providing the service?

Multiple choice questions

Directions for question 1: each of the questions or incomplete statements in this section is followed by five suggested answers. Select the best answer in each case.

Q1 Which of the following is *not* an enhanced service?

A   Supply of medicines via patient group directions
B   Medicines use review
C   Smoking-cessation services
D   Minor ailments schemes
E   Supervised administration of medicines

Directions for questions 2 and 3: for each numbered question select the one lettered option above it which is most closely related to it. Within each group of questions each lettered option may be used once, more than once, or not at all.

A   Pre-contemplation stage
B   Preparation stage
C   Action stage
D   Maintenance stage
E   Relapse

Q2 In a consultation in a smoking-cessation clinic the client acknowledges that there are certain dangers in smoking and has some thoughts about giving up smoking.
Q3 At this stage of the smoking-cessation programme the role of the pharmacist is to keep regular contact with the client and ensure that the client is motivated to continue with the programme.

Directions for questions 4 to 7: each of the questions or incomplete statements in this section is followed by three responses. For each question ONE or MORE of the responses is (are) correct. Decide which of the responses is (are) correct. Then choose:

A   if **1**, **2** and **3** are correct
B   if **1** and **2** only are correct
C   if **2** and **3** only are correct
D   if **1** only is correct
E   if **3** only is correct

Directions summarised:
A: 1, 2, 3   B: 1, 2 only   C: 2, 3 only   D: 1 only   E: 3 only

Q4   Examples of patient access to a minor ailments scheme include:

1   Any patient registered with a GP practice that is participating in the scheme presents in a pharmacy
2   A voucher scheme where a patient is issued with a voucher to access the scheme
3   Referral of the patient by another healthcare professional

Q5   Suggested quality indicators for a smoking-cessation service include:

1   Comparison of the 2-week quit rate with the PCT target
2   Provision of appropriate health-promotion material from the pharmacy
3   Annual review of standard operating procedures for this service

Q6   Which of the statements about needle and syringe equipment is (are) true?

1   A 0.5 ml insulin syringe is suitable for drug misusers who inject subcutaneously
2   If no good veins are present and the drug misuser is injecting intramuscularly a 25G, 16 mm needle would be suitable
3   Complaints from clients about the quality of the equipment are infrequent

Q7   In a supervised administration of methadone scheme the following is (are) true:

1   Sugar-free and colour-free products have less potential to be abused
2   The pharmacist should observe the client swallowing a drink of water directly after taking the methadone
3   To offer this service an agreement is set up between the prescriber, pharmacist, client and client's keyworker

Directions for questions 8 to 10: the following questions consist of a statement in the left-hand column followed by a second statement in the right-hand column.

Decide whether the first statement is true or false.

Decide whether the second statement is true or false.

Then choose:

A   if both statements are true and the second statement is a correct explanation of the first statement

B   if both statements are true but the second statement is NOT a correct explanation of the first statement

C   if the first statement is true but the second statement is false

D   if the first statement is false but the second statement is true

E   if both statements are false

Directions summarised:

A:	True	True	second statement is **a correct explanation** of the first
B:	True	True	second statement is **NOT a correct explanation** of the first
C:	True	False	
D:	False	True	
E:	False	False	

Q8

- *Statement 1*: The support service offered to care homes includes advice and support to residents and staff over and above the dispensing essential service.
- *Statement 2*: This support service can only be provided by a PCT-accredited pharmacist that regularly supplies the home with medication.

Q9

- *Statement 1*: Enhanced services are not part of the national pharmacy contract.
- *Statement 2*: Enhanced services are commissioned at a local level by primary care organisations.

Q10

- *Statement 1*: The crushing of tablets and capsules may present a health and safety risk to the person administering the dose.
- *Statement 2*: The crushing of tablets presents a legal issue as the product is being administered outside the product licence.

Case studies

Level 1

Lucy is a pharmacy undergraduate working on a summer placement in a community pharmacy that is offering a 'stop smoking' enhanced service. She is keen to find out more about the service and her tutor obtains consent from a new client for Lucy to observe their first meeting.

Lucy makes a note of the following background details on Client AB:

- 25-year-old female
- smoking since aged 16
- has come to clinic as a result of direct advertising at local health centre
- not taking any medication, no medical conditions
- overweight and has recently started to improve diet and take more exercise
- very keen to stop smoking and wants to become pregnant
- smokes approximately 20 cigarettes a day, does not have a cigarette on waking. Smokes quite a lot socially, especially at mealtimes and when out in the evening
- has not made a serious attempt to quit before, but appears well motivated to stop smoking
- shows some interest in using NRT gum.

What areas of discussion do you think Lucy's tutor should include in the first meeting with this client?

Level 2

Nick is a preregistration trainee in a community pharmacy that provides a medicines-management and advisory service to over 30 care homes. His tutor has just received a phone call from the manager of a nursing home about an elderly resident, Mrs Avril Rose, who has swallowing difficulties.

The home manager is trying to find out:

- if there are any liquid formulations that Mrs Rose could use instead of tablets
- if any of the tablets can be crushed or the capsules opened up before taking.

The preregistration tutor is very busy and arranges to call the care manager back later that day.

Patient medication record (PMR) for Mrs Avril Rose, Fairlawn Nursing Home, DOB 02/01/27

- Bendroflumethiazide 2.5 mg i om
- Ramipril 5 mg tablets i om
- Co-codamol 8/500 tablets i–ii qds prn
- Levothyroxine 50 mcg tablets i od
- Aspirin 75 mg tablets i od
- Senna tablets ii on
- Amoxicillin 500 mg caps i tds (7 days).

Nick is asked by his tutor to look at the PMR record for Mrs Rose and prepare a suitable answer that they can discuss together before the tutor returns the phone call.

- What would you advise Nick to include in his response?

Level 3

Meera is a local community pharmacist who also works part-time for the PCT. Currently there is some interest in providing minor ailments schemes through local pharmacies to relieve pressure on practice staff at local health centres. Meera is part of a PCT working group that consists of a GP, practice nurse, practice manager and another pharmacist.

The practice nurse can see some advantages of the scheme as it will release some of her time. The GP is concerned that there may be problems with communication of information about patients and duplication of effort. He is also concerned about quality issues and how the service would be monitored. The practice manager thinks a scheme should be piloted but is concerned over increasing amounts of administration. She expresses the view that the scheme may generate a lot more paperwork.

Meera has worked in a neighbouring PCT and has successfully managed a minor ailments scheme in the past. She is asked to present a short summary of her previous experience to present to the next meeting.

- What specific points do you think Meera should include in her presentation to address the concerns of her colleagues?

References

1   Department of Health. *Choosing Health through Pharmacy. A programme for pharmaceutical public health 2005–2015*. London: Department of Health, 2005. www.dh.gov.uk/en/Publicationsandstatistics/Publications /PublicationsPolicyAndGuidance/DH_4107494 (accessed 10 September 2007).
2   Celino G, Blenkinsopp A, Dhalla M. *Pharmaceutical Needs Assessment*

Toolkit. London: National Primary and Care Trust Development Programme, 2003.

3   National Pharmacy Association. *Commissioning Resource Pack.* St Albans: National Pharmacy Association, 2005.

4   Bradley F, Elvey R, Ashcroft D, Noyce P. Commissioning services and the new community pharmacy contract: pharmaceutical needs assessment and uptake of new pharmacy contracts. *Pharm J* 2006; **277**: 161–163.

5   Bradley F, Elvey R, Ashcroft D, Noyce N. Commissioning services and the new community pharmacy contract: (2) drivers, barriers and approaches to commissioning. *Pharm J* 2006; **277**: 189–192.

6   Bradley F, Kendall J, Ashcroft D *et al.* Setting up local pharmaceutical services – lessons for pharmacy contractors. *Pharm J* 2005; **274**: 548–551.

7   Bradley F, Elvey R, Ashcroft D, Noyce P. Commissioning services and the new community pharmacy contract: (3) uptake of enhanced services. *Pharm J* 2006; **277**: 224–226.

8   Pharmaceutical Services Negotiating Committee. *Enhanced Services Costing Toolkit.* www.psnc.org.uk/uploaded_txt/PCLS%20076.06%20 Enhanced%20Costing%20Toolkit%20Version%202.pdf (accessed 10 October 2007).

9   News item. Should benchmark prices be agreed for enhanced services in England? *Pharm J* 2006; **277**: 443.

10   Pharmaceutical Services Negotiating Committee. *Enhanced Service Speci-fication – Care Home (Support and Advice on Storage, Supply and Adminis-tration of Drugs and Appliances).* www.psnc.org.uk/uploaded_txt/EN5%20 -%20Care%20home%20support.pdf (accessed 10 September 2007).

11   Centre for Pharmacy Postgraduate Education. *Open Learning Course for Pharmacists. Supporting care homes with medicines management.* Manchester: Centre for Pharmacy Postgraduate Education.

12   Wright D. Tablet crushing is a widespread practice but it is not safe and may not be legal *Pharm J* 2002; **269**: 132.

13   Parrott S, Godfrey C, Raw M, West R, McNeill AD. Guidance for com-missioners on the cost-effectiveness of smoking cessation interventions. *Thorax* 1998; **53** (Suppl 5): S1–38.

14   McNeill A. Preventing the onset of tobacco use. In: Bolliger CT, Fagerstrom KO, eds. *The Tobacco Epidemic. Progress in repiratory research, 28.* Basel: Karger, 1997.

15   Department of Health. *Smoking Kills: a white paper on tobacco.* CM 4177. London: The Stationery Office, 1998.

16   Department of Health. *Statistics on NHS Stop Smoking Services in England, April 2004–March 2005.* London: Department of Health, 2005.

17   Bradley F, Elvey R, Ashcroft D, Noyce P. Commissioning services and the new community pharmacy contract: (3) Uptake of enhanced services. *Pharm J* 2006; **277**: 224–226.

18   Pharmaceutical Services Negotiating Committee. *NHS Community Phar-*

macy Contractual Framework. Enhanced service specification – stop smoking. www.psnc.org.uk/uploaded_txt/EN4%20-%20Stop%20Smoking.pdf (accessed 10 September 2007).

19   Prochaska J, DiClemente CC. The transtheoretical approach: crossing traditional boundaries of therapy. Melbourne, FL: Krieger, 1994.

20   Department of Health. *Building the Best – Choice, Responsiveness and Equity in the NHS.* London: Department of Health, 2003.

21   National Pharmacy Association. *Implementing a Community Pharmacy Minor Ailment Scheme. A practical toolkit for primary care organisations and health professionals.* London: National Pharmacy Association, 2003.

22   Vohra S. A community pharmacy minor ailment scheme – effective, rapid and convenient. *Pharm J* 2006; **276**: 754–756.

23   World Health Organization. *Effectiveness of Sterile Needle and Syringe Programming in Reducing HIV/AIDS among Injecting Drug Users.* Geneva: World Health Organization, 2004. www.emro.who.int/aiecf/web301.pdf (accessed 10 September 2007).

24   Parsons J, Hickman M, Turnbull PJ *et al.* Over a decade of syringe exchange: results from 1997 UK survey. *Addiction* 2002; **97**: 845–850.

25   Sheridan J, Strang J, Taylor C, Barber N. HIV prevention and drug treatment services for drug misusers: a national study of community pharmacists' attitudes and involvement in service specific training. *Addiction* 1997; **92**: 1737–1748.

26   Lawrie T, Matheson C, Bond CM, Roberts K. Pharmacy customers' views and experiences of using pharmacies which provide drug misuse services. *Drug Alcohol Review* 2004; **23**: 195–202.

27   Royal Pharmaceutical Society of Great Britain. *Medicines, Ethics and Practice. A guide for pharmacists and pharmacy technicians.* Number 31. London: Royal Pharmaceutical Society of Great Britain, 2007.

28   Kayne S. Methadone: a question of supervision. *Chemist and Druggist* 1996; **245**: VI–VII.

29   News item. ACMD calls for methadone supervision. *Pharm J* 2000; **265**: 6.

30   Royal Pharmaceutical Society of Great Britain. *e-PIC References on Supervised Administration of Methadone.* www.rpsgb.org.uk/pdfs/methadone.pdf (accessed 10 September 2007).

31   Newell G. Providing methadone services – case studies. *Pharm J* 2001; **266**: 542–546.

32   Centre for Pharmacy Postgraduate Education. Distance learning package. *Drug Use and Misuse.* London: Centre for Pharmacy Postgraduate Education.

33   Chaulk CP, Kazandjian VA. Directly observed therapy for treatment completion of pulmonary tuberculosis: consensus statement of the Public Health Tuberculosis Guidelines Panel. *Journal of the American Medical Association* 1998; **279**: 943–948.

Further information

Scott J, Bruce L. Practical advice on medical complications of intravenous drug misuse. *Pharm J* 1998; **260**: 957–960.

National Pharmacy Association. *Medicines in Care Homes. A training pack for pharmacists to use in the training of care home staff.* London: National Pharmacy Association, 2004.

7

Supplying medication

If in doubt, don't give it out!

(Anonymous)

Checkpoint

Before reading on, think about the following questions to identify your own knowledge gaps in this area:

- How is an accredited checking technician prepared for their role?
- What are some of the advantages of non-medical independent prescribing?
- Describe the stages involved in managing a dispensing error.

The supply of medication has always been a core role for the community pharmacist. The importance of the supply function is underlined by the definition of dispensing as an essential service in the pharmacy contract. However, as the community pharmacist moves towards more patient-centred services, the practical issues surrounding the supply function need to be examined more closely. This chapter aims to look at a range of key issues that impact on the pharmacist's role of supplying medication. Wide-ranging areas such as practical dispensary design, the integration of newer roles for support staff and different ways of accessing medication, such as patient group directions and pharmacist prescribing, are all discussed in this chapter.

Dispensary design and workflow

The ideal dispensary is tidy and clean with uncluttered work surfaces, a logical layout of dispensing stock and a natural workflow. The minimum standards for any dispensary include:

- a good basic standard of decoration for the walls, ceilings and all paintwork
- a cleanable floor

- adequate fixtures and fittings, uncluttered surfaces that are smooth and impervious to dirt and moisture
- a clean refrigerator that is regularly defrosted and contains a minimum/maximum thermometer
- clean sinks with both hot and cold water available
- the proper storage and disposal of waste materials.

Even when these basic minimum standards are met, there needs to be considerable thought about the way that the workflow of the dispensary is arranged to be able to offer an efficient and safe dispensing service. An example of efficient workflow in a pharmacy is outlined in Figure 7.1.

The cost of labour is by far the greatest cost in running a dispensary. With the potentially reduced involvement of the pharmacist in dispensing activities, the day-to-day management of the dispensary should ideally be delegated to a pharmacy technician. An efficient workflow has the following advantages:

- more economic and efficient use of labour
- reduced waiting times for patients
- increased time available for contact and interaction with patients
- less likelihood of dispensing errors
- more efficient stock-rotation procedures
- reduced frustration in an ordered working environment, resulting in increased staff morale.

The overall design of a dispensary should depend on the type of dispensing that is taking place. For example if there is a large proportion of repeat dispensing, there needs to be a large working area that is assigned to this activity. When considering the design of the dispensary and arrangement of stock it is useful to refer to the standard operating procedure (SOP) for dispensing. The SOP for dispensing will be specific for a pharmacy and should take into account any specific design features that impact on the dispensing process.

The dispensing process can be divided into seven stages:

1 prescription reception
2 legal and clinical check
3 labelling of item(s)
4 assembly of item(s)
5 checking of item(s)
6 final check
7 hand to patient/counselling.

Prescription reception

An efficient dispensing service is dependent on a clearly defined prescription-reception procedure. The area where prescriptions are

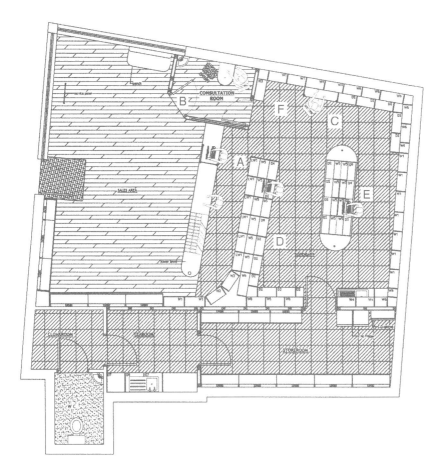

A   Pharmacist based 'front of house' to interact directly with clients. Pharmacist has access by laptop to patient medication records and a good view of the entire pharmacy. Any acute 'waiting' prescriptions are passed directly to the pharmacist for checking.

B   The client can walk into the consultation room easily from the shop floor to have a confidential conversation.

C   There is a clearly defined administration area (access to email, fax and telephone) where a designated member of staff can answer all queries relating to repeat prescriptions. A large area is available for filing paperwork.

D   Waiting prescription dispensing area.

E   Repeat prescription dispensing area.

F   Clear area for storage of prescriptions, out of view of the customer but close to the reception desk.

Figure 7.1   Example of a pharmacy design to allow efficient workflow. Plan reproduced with kind permission of Kevin Smith, community pharmacist, Harborough Field Pharmacy, Rushden and Crescent Installations Ltd.

handed in should be clear and unambiguous. Any support staff involved in this process must have been trained to a basic minimum level. Assisting in the supply of prescribed items, which involves taking in a prescription and issuing prescribed items, is part of the specific knowledge and understanding required for the Pharmacy Services Scottish/National Vocational Qualification (S/NVQ) level 2. To ensure a smooth prescription process the member of staff receiving a prescription should be able to:

- recognise different types of prescription form. The Prescription Pricing Division of the NHS Business Services Authority has a useful website that outlines all the different types of NHS prescription and the legal requirements for prescription writing:[1]
- ensure that the patient's name, including forename and address are legible
- establish if the prescription is being handed in by the patient or their representative
- verify the age of the patient if the prescription is for a child
- take any prescription charge that is due or deal with any exemption prescription queries. In practice this will mean that the member of staff should be able to recognise contraceptive items that are exempt from prescription charges and items that attract a multiple prescription charge, and be fully aware of the procedure for completing the back of the prescription form. Point-of-dispensing checks act as an important deterrent for patient fraud and have contributed to a 60% reduction in patient prescription fraud in recent years. It is vital that the member of staff receiving a prescription is fully aware of the procedures involved in checking exemption from prescription charges[2]
- access the patient medication record (PMR) system. It is useful if the member of staff can access the PMR system to confirm patient details, and change any administrative details such as address. Sometimes at this stage of the process a patient may ask a non-clinical question such as the timing of their repeat prescription. This type of query should be answered promptly without interrupting the dispensing process
- adopt a safe procedure when the prescription item can be purchased and costs less than a prescription charge. This will involve liaison with the pharmacist as this involves interpreting the prescription and prescriber's intentions
- determine the time it will take for the prescription to be dispensed and communicate this to the patient.

Some busy pharmacies prefer to use a numbered docket system when receiving prescriptions. This can be useful in areas where there are potential language difficulties. The SOP for prescription reception needs to take into account all of the above requirements.

Legal and clinical check

This part of the process must be performed by the pharmacist, preferably in an area free from distractions. Some of the legal checks may have already been carried out at the reception stage. For example the assistant may have spotted that the prescription is out of date or a repeat direction on a private prescription is invalid. It is important that any legal issues are confirmed by the pharmacist before communicating with the patient. Extra care needs to be taken with prescriptions for controlled drugs (CDs) to ensure that all legal requirements are satisfied. Once the pharmacist is satisfied that the prescription is legally valid they should proceed to the clinical check.

The clinical check involves interpreting the wishes of the prescriber and making a pharmaceutical assessment of the prescription. This involves checking the prescription for safety, quality and efficacy. A systematic protocol should be developed by the individual pharmacist covering such areas as:

- name, strength and form of the drug. Is it clear what is intended?
- what dose form is required?
- is the dose appropriate for the indication and age of patient? What type of dose has been prescribed – starting dose or maintenance dose?
- is it an intended unlicensed 'off-label' prescription
- are there any allergies, contraindications or possible interactions indicated on the PMR?
- is the formulation appropriate?
- is the quantity appropriate?

Any queries about the prescription should be highlighted at this stage and the prescriber contacted for further clarification or information. Any potential problems should be resolved before proceeding any further with the dispensing process. A vital role of the community pharmacist is to intercept problem prescriptions. One study demonstrated that nationally 280 000 potentially serious prescription errors are detected every year.[3]

The pharmacist is using their clinical and pharmaceutical knowledge to ensure that the patient receives the best possible pharmaceutical care and receives the correct drug in an appropriate formulation and dose. Barriers to this process are that the pharmacist is not always aware of the diagnosis and does not have access to the patient's medical records. In the case of problem prescriptions, the pharmacist should communicate directly with the prescriber and not delegate this task. Once the prescription has been validated by the pharmacist it can be passed to the dispensary team to complete the remaining stages of the supply process.

Labelling of item(s)

The location of the labelling equipment should ideally be in a specially designated area that is free of interruptions, as this part of the process requires considerable concentration. For accurate label production the following areas need to be considered:

- the patient's details such as the correct spelling of the name. It is necessary to check that any incorrect spelling is not being propagated from a previous PMR entry
- an awareness of drugs with similar names. Handwritten prescriptions are less common but if the prescription is handwritten the name of the drug needs to be looked at carefully. Similar names such as chlorpropamide/chlorpromazine or disopyramide/dipyridamole need particular attention
- when selecting repeat medication from a patient's PMR it is important to check carefully if there are any dose or quantity changes
- the additional cautionary labelling automatically added by the PMR will need to be checked
- the quantity of the product prescribed needs to be considered in relation to the pack sizes available and whether multiple labels are required
- if an active stock control system is in place on the PMR it will be necessary to check remaining stock levels
- any owing medication will need to be recorded and the appropriate documentation produced for the patient.

There should be provision in the SOP for an emergency procedure to dispense prescriptions without the PMR, in the event of a power failure or computing problems

Assembly of item(s)

Both the prescription and the labels should then be passed on so that the prescription items can be assembled. Many busy pharmacies have a system of clipping the labels to the prescription and placing the prescriptions in order. It is vital that items are selected and assembled from the original prescription and not the labels. This avoids repeating any errors made at the labelling stage. The layout of dispensary stock and the type of storage systems used will have a big impact on this part of the dispensing process. Purpose-designed sloping shelves with easier back filling will facilitate good stock rotation. Location of commonly used items near to the dispensary bench will result in a significant reduction in movement in the dispensary and increase efficiency. When designing a new dispensary, some thought needs to be given to the overall size of the dispensary. If the floor area is too large it can result in unnecessary walking to locate items. If the dispensary is too small and the stock is located in only a small area this can lead to dispensary congestion and slow down the assembly process.

Checking the item(s)

The member of staff who has assembled the product needs to carry out a careful check of the product and label against the prescription. Conscientious checking of the dispensing at this stage will result in a reduced number of problems at the final checking stage. It is good practice for the dispensing label to be initialled by the member of staff who performs this check. The completed item(s) and prescription should then be placed in the final checking area. In a high-volume dispensary each completed prescription should be placed in a suitable plastic container in readiness for the final check. This process ensures segregation of items from different prescriptions.

Final check

The final accuracy check should be carried out by either the pharmacist or the accredited checking technician (ACT). The mnemonic 'HELP' may be useful when a final check is being made to ensure that all the necessary checks have been made.[4] Help is an acronym for:

H: 'how much' has been dispensed (open all unsealed blister cartons to check the contents are of the correct product at the correct strength) and check that the correct leaflet is present
E: an 'expiry date' check
L: 'label' checks for the correct patient's name, the correct product name, the correct dose and the correct warning(s)
P: 'product' check to ensure that the correct medication and strength has been supplied.

A useful practice is to use a pencil to physically point to different parts of the label as the prescription is finally checked.

If there are any errors it is important that the problem is immediately recorded in the dispensing error record as a 'near miss' for future analysis. The management of dispensing errors is discussed later in this chapter. The final check should be carried out in a designated area of the dispensary, and ideally the person carrying out the final check should not have been involved in the dispensing process. If this separation of duties is not possible, it is useful to take a short mental break to separate the dispensing and checking process. It is good practice to initial the label to indicate that a check has taken place and identity the person carrying out the final check.

Hand to patient/counselling

It is surprisingly easy to hand out a prescription to the wrong person. This may be due to patients with similar names or because the patient has a problem with hearing when their name is called out. The safest system is to ask the patient to confirm another piece of information such as their address before handing across the prescription. At this final stage of the supply process, care and attention to detail is vital to ensure the correct prescription is handed to the right patient with appropriate information and counselling. Pharmacists have a legal obligation to provide a manufacturer's patient information leaflet (PIL) each time a medicine is sold or supplied.[5] However, the pharmacist should not let the PIL become a substitute for counselling but a means of providing supporting additional information.

The area where prescriptions are collected needs to be clearly defined and separate from the handing-in point. An established prescription-collection area provides a more logical work pattern. If the final checking and handing out form part of the same process, it is a useful practice to perform a final visual check as the items are packaged and handed to the patient.

If the patient is calling back for their prescription, it will need to be packaged and stored securely near to the prescription-collection area.

Completed prescriptions are normally stored alphabetically in a sealed bag with the accompanying prescription attached to the bag. Some pharmacies package each prescription in a polythene bag so that the items can be easily examined at the handing-out stage. Ideally the prescription should be handed out by the pharmacist. The patient or their representative should be offered the opportunity to ask any questions about their prescription. If the pharmacist is unable to hand out the prescription personally, the completed prescription can only be handed out under their supervision. It is important that the pharmacy team is aware of this requirement if the pharmacist has to temporarily leave the dispensing area. The pharmacist supervising the handing out of a previously completed prescription needs to be aware that although the item may have been dispensed and checked by another pharmacist there is a shared responsibility to ensure that the patient receives the correct item.

It is only through compliance with robust risk-management policies and safe systems of work that potential problems are minimised at each stage of the dispensing process.

Patient medication records

PMRs are subject to data protection legislation. The Data Protection Act 1998 covers all types of data-retrieval systems including paper records. The person to whom the data relate is called the data subject. In a pharmacy this will generally be patients but it may also be any information recorded about an individual such as a doctor or a pharmacy employee. The person who determines how and for what purposes the personal data are processed is called a data controller. The Act is administered by the data-protection commissioner who registers details of all data controllers. The eight data-protection principles require that personal data shall be:

1 obtained and processed fairly and lawfully and shall not be processed at all unless certain conditions are met
2 obtained and processed for, in ways compatible with, one or more lawful purposes
3 adequate, relevant and not excessive in relation to that purpose or purposes
4 accurate and kept up to date
5 kept for no longer than necessary
6 processed in accordance with the rights of data subjects under the Act. These rights include:
   – inform the data subject if personal data are being processed
   – give data subjects a description of the data being processed, for what purposes and to whom they will be disclosed
   – provide data subjects with that information in an intelligible form within 40 days of the request
7 protected against unauthorised or unlawful processing and against accidental loss, destruction or damage
8 not transferred outside the European Economic Area (EEA) unless the recipient country operates the same controls on data protection as apply with the EEA.

All personal data used in pharmacy practice are classed as sensitive personal data, but explicit patient consent to keep PMRs is not deemed necessary.[6] However, it should be emphasised that all personnel who may process such data are bound by the pharmacist's duty of confidentiality. The pharmacy practice leaflet is often used to advise patients that PMRs are maintained in the pharmacy and are subject to confidentiality and access rights. It should be clear to the patient that they may request in writing to see their PMR, and for a charge may have a printed copy. Further guidance on the detail of complying with requests from data subjects is outlined in documentation from the Royal Pharmaceutical Society of Great Britain (RPSGB) Fitness to Practise and Legal Affairs Directorate.[7]

  If a patient asks for their PMR to be removed it would be necessary for the pharmacist to explain to the patient the positive benefits of keeping a full and accurate record in order to check previous medication, dose changes and interactions. If the patient was insistent about deleting the record, the pharmacist would need to make a professional decision as this would breach the NHS terms of service relating to providing a dispensing service.

The RPSGB *Medicines, Ethics and Practice* guide (MEP) specifies that the PMR system must:[8]

- be notified to the data protection commissioner
- incorporate access control mechanisms to minimise the risk of unauthorised or unnecessary access to patient-specific data
- have the facility to identify drug interactions and be able to highlight those that are potentially hazardous
- provide for the collection, storage and display of PMRs containing the following as a minimum:
  - sufficient information about the patient to allow accurate identification
  - the identity of the patient's general practitioner (GP)
  - the prescription details (quantity supplied, directions, date of dispensing and any balance owed).

Some PMR systems have the facility to link patient information to the documentation required for pharmacy services. For example, most of the details required on a medicines use review (MUR) form can be transferred directly from the PMR to produce a record in electronic format. Enhanced services such as a smoking-cessation service, where it is necessary to record each meeting with the client, can also be recorded using the PMR system. As part of the clinical governance framework, all clinically significant interventions and associated advice should be recorded.

If the pharmacist is in the position to select a new PMR system a trial of different systems should be undertaken to assess:

- ease of use for all team members
- ability to use shortcuts for speedy labelling
- facility to record additional information and appropriate prompts
- a clear link with the contractual framework and provision of different services.

Accredited checking technician

Accuracy checking of dispensing by pharmacy technicians has been the norm in many hospitals for some time. The role of the accredited checking technician (ACT) in community pharmacy is relatively new. Typically a pharmacy technician is selected for ACT training and accreditation by matching with specific criteria, such as:

- performance in the workplace and nomination by the pharmacist manager
- minimum period of time of post-NVQ3 qualification
- minimum amount of dispensary experience and time in their current role.

These time periods vary and are set by the accrediting organisation. The role of the ACT will not be suitable for all pharmacy technicians as personal qualities such as commitment, enthusiasm and willingness to take on additional responsibility need to be considered.

The introductory taught component of ACT training usually consists of a 2-day course covering specific aspects such as:

- legal and professional aspects
- packaging and labelling requirements
- SOPs
- risk management
- principles of how to check
- counselling skills.

Practical training will consist of checking a number of prescriptions that are subsequently rechecked by the supervising pharmacist. For example the technician may be required to check 1500 items over a minimum of 3 months, with the completion of a weekly reflective log to highlight problem prescriptions. During this practical training period if the technician makes any checking error, they will have to start again at the beginning of checking the 1500 items. Some training schemes allow for a small number of designated very minor errors during this process. Once the practical training has been completed successfully the technician is required to sit a practical examination, which consists of 40 to 50 dispensed items where they need to find all the errors. On satisfactory completion of this examination the technician undergoes a probationary period where a further 200 items have to be checked by the technician under normal dispensary conditions and rechecked by the pharmacist. The accreditation process involves considerable input and support from the supervising pharmacist both during and after training. This time commitment and the impact on the pharmacy team needs to be planned carefully. There is no further formal assessment once the technician is accredited. In order to ensure that standards are maintained, any specific issues need to be addressed through continuing professional development.

It is expected that the ACT will work closely with the pharmacist and take on a more significant management role within the dispensary to ensure that the team works within the agreed dispensing SOPs. The ACT role within community pharmacy has significant implications in terms of enabling the pharmacist to engage in newer ways of working.

Dispensing errors

Occasionally there can be a breakdown in the defence net of procedures to ensure that the right patient receives the right medicine. When a dispensing error occurs, everyone involved is likely to feel anxiety over the consequences of making an error.

In recent years there has been a move towards a more open culture and a transparent approach when dealing with errors and failures within the NHS. A special health authority, The National Patient Safety Agency (NPSA) was established in 2001 to co-ordinate national efforts of reporting errors and learning from mistakes and problems that affect patient safety.[9]

There are three areas to consider when managing a dispensing error:

- dealing with the error
- making a record
- reviewing the error.

Dealing with the error

In the event of a dispensing error there are three main reasons why complaints are made to the RPSGB.

- the fact that an error has been made at a pharmacy, which many members of the public believe should work at 100% accuracy
- the patient has been harmed by the error and may be contemplating a claim for compensation
- the patient or relative is dissatisfied with the way that the complaint was dealt with at the pharmacy.

When a dispensing error or adverse incident occurs, the fundamental rule is that the complaint should be managed in a professional manner that demonstrates that the matter is being taken seriously. Provided no harm has been done to the patient and the complaint is dealt with appropriately by the pharmacy, it is unlikely that the patient will take their complaint to an independent body such as the RPSGB or primary care trust (PCT).

If the patient has been issued with the wrong medicine it should be established at an early stage if they have taken any of the medicine. If the patient has taken any wrong medicine it is essential that this is treated as an immediate priority. The patient's GP should be contacted with a full explanation of what has been taken, the dosage and for how long. In more serious cases a label may have been transposed and the patient taken a high dose of the wrong medication. In this type of case it may be necessary to contact a local drug information centre for advice. The GP should always be informed if incorrect medication has been taken, even if no harm appears to have been caused.

Top tips for dealing with a dispensing error

- Do not delegate this important and sensitive task.
- Deal with the patient in a professional manner.
- Do not be defensive or try to minimise the error in any way.
- It is irrelevant to the patient that the error was not made by you personally.
- Do not be afraid to make an apology if it is a genuine error. If necessary, apologise on behalf of the pharmacist who has made the error.
- Explain that a full investigation will be made into the cause of the error.

The incorrect medication should be examined and full details of the error recorded. This information is vital for future review and analysis of the error. If the patient is willing for the pharmacist to retain the incorrect medication, this should be stored securely for a reasonable period of time, in case the incident develops further. The patient should not feel pressure to hand in the incorrect medication and may wish to retain the medicine personally. For safety reasons it would be useful to suggest that the medicine could be held securely by an independent body such as the RPSGB or PCT. The original prescription should be retrieved from the file or a copy of the prescription requested from the Prescription Pricing Division (PPD) as soon as possible.

The pharmacist must make it clear that a full internal investigation will be made into the cause of error and that the incident will be reported to the superintendent pharmacist. The correct medication that has been ordered on the original prescription should be promptly supplied to the patient.

If the patient has not been harmed in any way, the pharmacist will need to establish what the patient's expectation is from the pharmacy. For example if they expect some form of compensation it is important that the superintendent pharmacist is informed and it is clear that the patient will be contacted by the company. It is inadvisable to talk in specific terms about compensation until a full investigation has been made.

If the patient feels that an apology and internal investigation is inadequate and they wish to take their complaint further to an official body there are two options:

- provide the name and address of the RPSGB Fitness to Practise and Legal Affairs Directorate
- explain to the patient that they may wish to use the NHS complaints procedure and provide details of the local PCT. Further details of this are provided in the next section of this chapter.

If it appears likely that the complaint will be taken further, the pharmacist should check if there are any special conditions with their professional indemnity insurers, who will need to be informed if the patient intends to make a claim.

Making a record

A pharmacy incident action form or similar documentation should be used to record all of the details relating to the incident. A copy of the original prescription should be attached to the form. The form should include as much detail as possible to assist the review process and aim to prevent the same incident re-occurring. For example the precise time of the incident can provide important information about the working conditions in the pharmacy at the time. A copy of this document should be forwarded to the superintendent pharmacist. The patient should be given the opportunity to comment on the circumstances surrounding the incident, personnel involved and any other information that they consider to be relevant. Ideally an electronic copy of this form should be forwarded to the superintendent pharmacist as soon as possible after the pharmacist has become aware of the incident.

Reviewing the error

All errors should be subject to a review process irrespective of whether it is a 'near miss' identified at the final check stage or a dispensing error identified by a patient. A full and frank discussion of the circumstances leading up to the error is needed to highlight what factors may have contributed to the incident. This process enables the pharmacy team to have a greater understanding of why the error occurred and how it could be prevented in the future. The extent of the review will depend on the seriousness of the error and actual or potential harm caused to the patient. A root cause analysis is a method of investigating why things went wrong and how this may be prevented in the future.

Root cause analysis

A root cause analysis (RCA) should be carried out by a small group of staff who are familiar with the working practices of the dispensary. The RCA involves the following five stages:

1 information gathering

2 identification of the problem. This involves stating the actual problem such as the wrong drug has been supplied and then repeatedly asking 'Why?' until it becomes difficult to find an answer. This method is often called the 'Five whys', and after answering the why question several times the root cause of the problem is often established
3 identification of contributing factors. Accidents and errors can generally be traced back to one of five root causes: people, materials, environment, method or tools
4 propose and implement solutions to prevent the same error occurring again
5 complete a pharmacy risk-assessment tool which provides a working document to work towards future improvement (an example of a pharmacy risk-assessment tool is provided on the National Pharmacy Association (NPA) website).

The NPSA provides useful further information on root cause analysis.[10]

Errors can be categorised into the following types:[11]

■ there is an adequate procedure in place but the procedure is not followed out as intended:
  – *example*: the chloramphenicol eye drops are placed on the main dispensary shelves and not in the fridge
■ there is a lapse either in memory or concentration:
  – *example*: the pharmacy technician is interrupted by a trainee dispensing assistant in the middle of a large and complex prescription, and makes a labelling error
■ a 'rule based' error where knowledge is applied incorrectly or incompletely
  – *example*: a pharmacist performing the final check adds the incorrect expiry date to the label of an antibiotic mixture, believing that the expiry date is 14 days.

It is also possible that the error has been caused by a violation where a member of staff has not adhered to an existing SOP or protocol. For example, during a busy dispensing period a trainee may not have known a dosage code on the PMR and decided to free type a dispensing label, resulting in erroneous instructions. The pharmacist undertaking the final check may not have been systematic and not have thoroughly checked the label. This error is a result of both the dispensing assistant and the pharmacist not following established procedures. When discussing errors, the team needs to take a broad view using a number of headings. Suggested areas to consider could include:

■ pharmacy conditions
■ team members
■ systems and procedures.

Pharmacy conditions

When considering the pharmacy conditions it is useful to ask such questions as:

- is there any unnecessary noise or distraction in the dispensary?
- do the dispensary lighting, heating and working conditions meet the required standards?
- are there any non-dispensing tasks that are carried out in the dispensary?
- is the workspace uncluttered?
- is the dispensary well laid out with a logical workflow?
- is the equipment adequate? For example has a problem with a piece of equipment such as a tablet counter or labelling device contributed to an error?
- what is the breakdown and frequency of the workload at the time of the error? The PMR can provide this useful information which may determine 'danger' periods during the day. It is surprising that most dispensing errors do not take place during busy dispensing periods but are more likely following a break or during a quieter period. This may be associated with the lapse in concentration that can occur if a member of staff is not fully occupied with the task and may become distracted.

Team members

Factors to consider when considering the impact of the team are:

- the health of the team such as any problems that may have affected their concentration. This issue could range from eyesight problems and the need for regular eye tests to a member of staff being ill at the time of the incident. Good hearing is also a consideration, as much communication in a pharmacy is by telephone
- if any members of the team were tired or have been working for too long on a particular task
- communication or conflict issues within the team that could impact on the dispensing process
- distraction issues caused by personal problems
- competence of staff members to undertake dispensing duties. If staff competence is an issue then this needs to be examined as a wider performance-management issue
- staff working patterns such as under- or over-staffing and pharmacist lone working.

Systems and procedures

All parts of the dispensing process need to be reviewed and it is likely that the error will shift the focus of the review on to a specific part of the process. Typical areas that need to be considered include:

- incorrect interpretation of the prescription. Safe procedures should be in place in the event of a prescription being difficult to read. For example a colleague should always be asked to interpret a difficult prescription independently rather than being asked to confirm the interpretation of another team member. This process avoids the possibility of being influenced by any incorrect preconceived ideas

- labelling errors such as incorrect dosage instructions, transposing labels or selection of the wrong strength or wrong preparation from the PMR when repeating a label
- incorrect picking of medicines, for example the issue of drugs with similar names, or generic items with similar packaging. It may be necessary to review the way that certain stock items are laid out in order to minimise this type of error. For example a slow release form may have been incorrectly selected as it is in a very similar package to the usual form of the medication
- giving out the wrong prescription to the wrong patient. This may be due to an oversight when the items have been placed in a bag and the wrong details attached to the bag. It may be that the patient's address has not been checked properly at the time of handing out the prescription
- supplying out-of-date or contaminated stock due to poor stock-management processes
- incorrect owings procedure where stock is dispensed from an incorrect owings slip rather than the original prescription
- a problem with a product that has been prepared extemporaneously. This may be due to problems of technical competence or accuracy checking, or the problem may result from unsuitable premises and equipment.

As the prime concern of the pharmacist is the welfare of the patient, it is vital that adequate time is taken when an error takes place to discover precisely what went wrong. As part of overall clinical governance the steps taken to prevent the error from re-occurring and the accountable person for each action should be clearly documented on the pharmacy incident action form.

Electronic transmission of prescriptions

The overall aim of electronic transmission of prescriptions (ETP) is to replace the existing prescription system where the GP writes the prescription and the patient takes it to a pharmacy where it is dispensed and sent to the PPD for payment, with a totally electronic system. It is anticipated that once this basic process has been demonstrated to work, ETP will also be applied to repeat prescribing and medicines-management schemes.[12] Different pilot studies of ETP are being evaluated to look at the practicalities of what is expected to be a radical change in the way that medicine is prescribed in the UK.

Pilot schemes include:

- a relay or 'pull' model which allows patients to have complete freedom of choice as to where their prescription is dispensed. The prescription is sent by the GP to a central server and then downloaded when the patient goes to a pharmacy of their choice. A copy of the prescription is then sent to the PPD

- a 'push' or direct transmission to pharmacies model where the patient nominates a specific pharmacy to receive their electronic prescriptions. This system could include patients ordering home delivery of prescriptions and repeat prescriptions via the internet
- a hybrid model that uses a push model for repeat prescriptions that are sent directly to the patient's nominated pharmacy. Acute prescriptions would take the form of a barcode that holds prescription data and a digital signature.

A study into the benefits and barriers in implementing a system for ETP in the NHS suggests a number of possible benefits and barriers to the introduction of ETP.[13]

Possible benefits are:

- fewer medication and transcription errors
- increased efficiency
- better communication channels
- fraud reduction
- repeat prescribing benefits
- decreased costs
- improved prescription quality – for example improved compliance with legal requirements as a prescriber is prompted to complete the prescription
- improved practice and public health as more time is spent directly on patient care.

Possible barriers are:

- potential threat to privacy and security
- cultural and organisation issues surrounding the way that doctors and pharmacists work
- senior management and clinician commitment
- cost of transformation
- legal issues such as the area of controlled drugs
- technical problems such as computer failure
- education and implementation issues
- professional, practice and patient issues, for example concerns over less time for the patient with the doctor, the effect on small high street pharmacies, and the patient's perspective of electronic prescribing.

Managing customer complaints about NHS services

If a customer wishes to make a formal complaint about pharmacy services, the pharmacist is required to have a procedure in place for dealing with complaints about NHS services. The procedure should be in writing and be in line with the NHS (Complaints) Regulations 2004.[14] Customers should be informed of the complaints procedure in the pharmacy practice leaflet. Formal complaints are relatively rare and many expressions of concern do not necessarily lead to a complaint if handled correctly. All frontline members of the pharmacy team should be fully aware of the procedures in place and involve the pharmacist in any conversation at the earliest opportunity.

The pharmacy contractor should appoint a complaints manager who has responsibility for ensuring that the complaints procedure is followed correctly. The complaints manager is often the pharmacy manager but may also be another experienced member of staff. The complaint can be received either orally or in writing. In the case of an oral complaint a written record should be made. A suitable form can be downloaded from the Pharmaceutical Services Negotiating Committee (PSNC) website.[15] The relevant details recorded should include:

- name of the person complaining (the person presenting the complaint may be a patient or their representative)
- the nature of the complaint
- the date of the complaint.

If the complaint is in writing, the complaints manager should make a record of the date the complaint was received. All forms and documentation should be stored in a confidential filing system.

For a complaint to be investigated under the NHS procedure, there is a 6-month timeframe for the complainant to present the complaint. On receipt of written complaint a written acknowledgement should be sent within two working days of the date on which it was received. If the complaint was made orally a written acknowledgement should also be made within two working days and a copy of the written record made at the time of the complaint. The letter of acknowledgement should inform the complainant of the right to be assisted by the Independent Complaints Advocacy Service (ICAS). This is a body set up by the Department of Health to support patients or their carers complaining about NHS services.

The complaint should be investigated in the pharmacy using normal procedures such as interviewing staff and checking prescription records. This process will depend on the nature and seriousness of the complaint. If the complaint is legitimate a root cause analysis should be carried out. The complainant should be informed of the progress of the investigation and a record of all communication should be logged. It is useful at this stage if the complaints manager can obtain some indication from the complainant of what their expectation is in terms of acceptance of an apology or whether they are considering taking legal action.

Having completed the investigation, a response should be sent in writing within 25 working days of the date in which the complaint was made. The response should include:

- a summary of the complaint
- a summary of the investigation
- an indication of any changes in procedure in the pharmacy as a result of the complaint
- the right of the patient to refer the complaint to the Healthcare Commission
- another reminder of the right to be assisted by ICAS.

In the event of a more serious complaint, it is necessary to seek advice on drafting the response from the pharmacist's professional indemnity insurance agents. The response letter should be signed by either the pharmacy contractor or the senior manager if the pharmacy is within a multiple group.

Patient group directions

Historically patient group directions (PGDs) developed from a need to provide patient-focused services. In many cases the need to have a prescription signed often hindered the supply and administration process. For example nurses running a travel or child immunisation clinic often used a 'group protocol' to speed up the process of obtaining individual prescriptions. Group protocols were formally acknowledged and clarified in law in 2000 when the name changed to patient group directions.

The legal definition of a PGD is:

A written instruction for the sale, supply and/or administration of named medicines in an identified clinical situation.

It applies to groups of patients who may not be individually identified before presenting for treatment.

The PGD provides a legal framework which allows certain healthcare professionals to supply and administer medicines to groups of patients who fit the criteria laid out in the PGD. This means that a healthcare professional could supply and/or administer a medicine directly to a patient without the need for a prescription or an instruction from an individual prescriber. Using a PGD is not a form of prescribing, as it only allows the supply and administration of specified medicines to patients who fall into a defined group that is specified within the PGD documentation. The patient presents directly to the healthcare professional using the PGD without seeing a doctor. It is the responsibility of the healthcare professional working within the PGD to ensure that the patient fits the criteria set out in the PGD.

A PGD has the following characteristics:

- it is more applicable to services where the medicines supply follows a predictable pattern
- it is more appropriate for specific treatment episodes
- it is not intended for long-term care.

The production and authorisation of a PGD involves a multidisciplinary group that includes a doctor, pharmacist and a senior representative of the professional group using the PGD. A PGD for use in a community pharmacy must be authorised by the local PCT. In practice this will mean that the documentation must be signed by a doctor and pharmacist, approved by the PCT prescribing management group and authorised by the PCT clinical governance lead. The individual pharmacist who will be using the PGD must be named and authorised with appropriate signed documentation.

There are a number of professional groups who are able to use PGDs. Unlike prescribing where the healthcare professional requires additional formal qualifications, there is no such requirement for a PGD. However the PCT has a responsibility to ensure that the healthcare professional is assessed as competent and is a registered member of their profession acting within their code of conduct. There is a competency framework for healthcare professionals using PGDs. The competency framework is divided into three main areas:

- the consultation which includes clinical and pharmaceutical knowledge, establishing options for treatment and communicating with patients
- effective supply and administration with a PGD which includes safe PGD use, professional standards and practice development
- PGDs in context which includes accessing relevant information, understanding local and national policies and the ability to work both in a team and alone for the benefit of patients.

Full details of this competency framework are provided in the National Prescribing Centre documentation.[16]

Pharmacists are ideally placed to offer this type of service and there are many examples of PGDs used in a pharmacy such as nicotine-replacement products, anti-obesity medication and emergency hormonal contraception. Standard prescription charge rules and exemptions apply to all patients receiving a supply of medicines under a PGD from the NHS. This can sometimes be to the advantage of the patient and improve patient accessibility. For example the supply of a nicotine-replacement product, when the prescription charge will be considerably less than the cost of the item.

A PGD is very similar to the procedure used when making a sale and following a formal protocol. Provision of medication under a PGD opens up new possibilities for the community pharmacist interested in offering enhanced services and improved choice for the patient.

Pharmacists as prescribers

It is important to distinguish between supplementary prescribing and independent prescribing.

Supplementary prescribing is defined as a voluntary partnership between the independent prescriber (a doctor or a dentist) and a supplementary prescriber to implement an agreed patient-specific clinical management plan (CMP), with the patient's agreement.[17] In April 2003 the government enabled nurses and pharmacists to train to become supplementary prescribers. The nurse and pharmacist supplementary prescribers are able to prescribe any medicine including CDs and unlicensed medicines that are listed in the agreed CMP. Supplementary prescribers may prescribe for any medical condition provided their prescribing complies with the terms of the CMP agreed with the doctor.

In 2005 a joint Department of Health/Medicines and Healthcare products Regulatory Agency consultation looked at the option of independent prescribing by nurses. Around the same time there was a consultation on the possibility of independent prescribing by pharmacists. Consideration of both consultations resulted in changes in the regulations from May 2006 to enable suitably trained nurses and pharmacists to qualify as independent prescribers.

Independent prescribing can be defined as prescribing by a practitioner who is responsible and accountable for the assessment of patients with undiagnosed or diagnosed conditions and for decisions about the clinical management required, including prescribing. An independent prescriber will be able to prescribe any licensed medicine for any medical condition that they are competent to treat. At the time of writing, pharmacist independent prescribers cannot prescribe CDs. Nurse independent prescribers can prescribe a limited range of CDs as specified by the *Drug Tariff* for specific medical conditions. Further information on pharmacist and nurse prescribing is provided on the PSNC website.[18]

A pharmacist independent prescriber must be registered with the RPSGB with an annotation signifying that the pharmacist has qualified as an independent prescriber. This involves the successful completion of a training programme accredited by the RPSGB. The pharmacist must have had at least 2 years' practice experience in a clinical environment in either a hospital or a community setting. If a pharmacist is considering independent prescribing they should be able to demonstrate competence to prescribe in the area in which they will prescribe following training. A scoping and support guide that includes generic competencies for pharmacists involved in prescribing is available from the National Prescribing Centre.[19] Apart from the advantage of improved patient access and choice of a prescriber, the introduction of non-medical independent prescribing should also encourage team working across the NHS. It is important that prescribing is carried out within a multidisciplinary team where there is access to a single healthcare record.

Pharmacists who wish to train as prescribers would normally need to:

- establish a prescribing partnership with a medical practitioner
- obtain the agreement of their local PCT that pharmacist independent prescribing will meet a local service need. This means that it will improve patient access or meet local health targets
- apply to the local Workforce Development Confederation for funding of a training programme.

Pharmacist supplementary prescribers who have been qualified as a prescriber for less than 5 years can become independent prescribers by completing a conversion course. The conversion course involves both formal training and supervision by a medical practitioner. The conversion course is designed to develop decision-making skills in terms of clinical assessment. The prescriber must be competent to refer the patient if they have other conditions that need further investigation.

As there is no CMP, independent pharmacist prescribing may be useful in a number of different situations. Examples of potential pharmacist involvement in independent prescribing include:

- prescribing starting doses more easily and efficiently
- continuing care of the patient where the CMP has not yet been prepared and established
- situations such as when the patient has swallowing difficulties and there needs to be a substitution with a different product form. Independent prescribing would allow rapid treatment without waiting for authorisation from a doctor
- pharmacokinetic scenarios where the pharmacist is well qualified to manage patient care and communicate best practice within the medical team
- running specialist clinics such as anticoagulation clinics
- filling geographical or skills gaps in services
- meeting the needs of patients who find it hard to access services, such as housebound patients
- management of long-term conditions such as hypertension
- management of co-morbidities and complex medication regimes.

The independent pharmacist prescriber is well placed to offer accessible and innovative services to the patient.

The NHS Plan emphasised the need to arrange and deliver services around the needs of patients.[20] The focus on the needs of patients and more flexible working by healthcare professionals continues to be an important emphasis.[21] One area that is particularly relevant to the community pharmacist is the demand for increased choice of where, when and how to get medicines. Increasingly the pharmacist will need to engage in different ways of meeting the medication needs of patients.

Implications for practice

Activity 1

- Take a critical look at your dispensary. Are there any changes that could be made to improve workflow and the efficiency of the dispensing process?

Activity 2

- Carry out a short study of any dispensing 'near misses' that have occurred over the past 6 months. Summarise the types of error that have been recorded and discuss with your pharmacy team how these can be avoided in the future.

Multiple choice questions

Directions for questions 1: each of the questions or incomplete statements in this section is followed by five suggested answers. Select the best answer.

Q1   Which of the following is a standard specified in the RPSGB *Professional Standards for the Sale and Supply of Medicines*?

A   Dispensary flooring that is impervious to dirt and moisture
B   A fridge that contains a maximum/minimum thermometer
C   Dispensary shelves that can be enclosed and locked
D   Dispensing benches that are height adjustable
E   A clean sink that has a mixer tap connected to hot and cold water

Directions for questions 2 to 3: for each numbered question select the one lettered option above it which is most closely related to it. Within each group of questions each lettered option may be used once, more than once, or not at all.

A   Prescription reception
B   Legal and clinical check
C   Assembly of prescription
D   Final check
E   Handing to patient

Q2   This part of the dispensing process can only be carried out by a
         pharmacist.
Q3   This part of the dispensing process can only be carried out by a
         pharmacist or accredited checking technician.

Directions for questions 4 to 7: each of the questions or incomplete
statements in this section is followed by three responses. For each question ONE or MORE of the responses is (are) correct. Decide which of the
responses is (are) correct. Then choose:

A   if **1**, **2** and **3** are correct
B   if **1** and **2** only are correct
C   if **2** and **3** only are correct
D   if **1** only is correct
E   if **3** only is correct

Directions summarised:
A: 1, 2, 3   B: 1, 2 only   C: 2, 3 only   D: 1 only   E: 3 only

Q4   Data-protection principles require that personal data shall be:

1   Accurate and kept up to date
2   Kept for no longer than necessary
3   Provided to data subjects within 40 days of written request

Q5   All PMR systems must:

1   Be able to identify drug interactions
2   Be notified to the data-protection commissioner
3   Be able to transfer patient details to a medicine use review form

Q6   Training of an accredited checking technician usually involves:

1   The compilation of a practical portfolio of checking a large number of
         prescription items
2   A probationary period under the supervision of a pharmacist
3   A written examination

Q7   For good practice a record should be made in the pharmacy of:

1   All dispensing errors
2   All 'near misses'
3   The time and date of all dispensing incidents

Directions for questions 8 to 10: the following questions consist of a statement in the left-hand column followed by a second statement in the right-hand column.

Decide whether the first statement is true or false.

Decide whether the second statement is true or false.

Then choose:

A   if both statements are true and the second statement is a correct explanation of the first statement

B   if both statements are true but the second statement is NOT a correct explanation of the first statement

C   if the first statement is true but the second statement is false

D   if the first statement is false but the second statement is true

E   if both statements are false

Directions summarised:

A:	True	True	second statement is **a correct explanation** of the first
B:	True	True	second statement is **NOT a correct explanation** of the first
C:	True	False	
D:	False	True	
E:	False	False	

Q8

- *Statement 1*: The pharmacy contractor should appoint a complaints manager who has responsibility for ensuring that the complaints procedure is followed correctly.
- *Statement 2*: The complaints procedure for a community pharmacy should be in line with the NHS (Complaints) Regulations 2004.

Q9

- *Statement 1*: There is a requirement for the healthcare professional supplying a medicine using patient group directions to have an additional prescribing qualification.
- *Statement 2*: The primary care organisation has a responsibility to ensure that the healthcare professional using patient group directions is assessed as competent and is acting within their professional code of conduct.

Q10

- *Statement 1*: The pharmacist and nurse supplementary prescriber are able to prescribe any medicine including controlled drugs and unlicensed medicines that are listed in the agreed clinical management plan.
- *Statement 2*: Supplementary prescribers may prescribe for any medical condition provided their prescribing complies with the terms of the clinical management plan agreed with a doctor.

Level 1

Carla is a pharmacy undergraduate working in a community pharmacy on a summer placement. Today an elderly customer became agitated and angry when she asked him to confirm his address when he was handing in his prescription. The SOP for the receipt of a prescription from a new patient states that a check must be made to ensure that the patient details are correct. Carla tried to explain to the patient that the pharmacy would keep a record of his medicines and she wanted to ensure that his record was accurate. This information did not reassure the patient but seemed to make him more aggressive. He said that he had not given his permission for the pharmacy to keep records and did not want his personal details on a computer. He demanded to speak to the pharmacist.

- How do you think the pharmacist should respond to this patient?

Level 2

It was an extremely busy morning in the community pharmacy where Neil was working as a preregistration trainee. A locum pharmacist had been employed for the day as Neil's tutor was out of the pharmacy visiting residential homes. It was nearly lunchtime when Neil was approached by a regular customer Mr Jones, who passed across a packet of atenolol 100 mg tablets that had been dispensed earlier that morning. Mr Jones was concerned as the packet of tablets 'looked different and not the usual colour'. Neil saw immediately that a box of atenolol 100 mg tablets had been dispensed and labelled 'atenolol 50 mg tablets'. All other details on the label appeared to be correct. Mr Jones had not taken any of the medication as he wanted to check first to see if there had been a mistake. Neil asked the locum pharmacist to speak to Mr Jones.

The locum was aware of the increasing queue of customers building up and had overheard the conversation between Neil and Mr Jones. He took the packet of tablets from Neil and went into the dispensary. The locum then quickly peeled off the dispensing label and attached it to a packet of atenolol 50 mg tablets. He put the atenolol 100 mg tablets on the dispensary shelf; handed the relabelled tablets to Mr Jones and apologised for any inconvenience. Mr Jones started to examine the tablets carefully and before he was able to comment the pharmacist had called the next customer forward. Neil was very uneasy about this incident and decided to discuss this with his tutor the next day.

- After hearing Neil's version of events, Neil's tutor asked him what he would have done differently. How should the locum pharmacist have responded to this situation?

Level 3

Mike manages a small independent pharmacy that dispenses about 2500 NHS items a week from a crowded and inadequate dispensary. The proprietor has recently purchased the vacant shop next door to the pharmacy and intends to double the floor area and develop the pharmacy business. Mike has worked in the pharmacy for over 3 years and is well settled in the local community. The customers are mainly elderly and Mike has developed a very successful repeat prescription collection and delivery service. Mike is keen to develop new services and supply residential homes but currently does not have sufficient space. The proprietor would like Mike's input into the planning of the new premises.

- What suggestions would you give to the proprietor of this business?

References

1   NHS Business Services Authority, Prescription Pricing Division *Prescribers and FP10 Prescriptions*. www.ppa.org.uk/education/fp10. htm#link8 (accessed 11 September 2007).
2   Pharmaceutical Services Negotiating Committee. *Point of Dispensing Checks Guidance*. www.psnc.org.uk/index.php?type=more_news&id= 2406 (accessed 11 September 2007).
3   Greene R. Survey of prescription anomalies in community pharmacies: (1) prescription monitoring. *Pharm J* 1995; **254**: 476–481.
4   Royal Pharmaceutical Society of Great Britain. *Fitness to Practise and Legal Affairs Directorate Fact Sheet: eleven. Dealing with dispensing errors.* (Reviewed March 2006) www.rpsgb.org/pdfs/factsheet11.pdf (accessed 11 September 2007).
5   Royal Pharmaceutical Society of Great Britain. *Fitness to Practise and Legal Affairs Directorate Fact Sheet: three. The medicines for human use (marketing authorisation etc) Regulations 1994, and the effect thereof.* www.rpsgb.org/pdfs/factsheet3.pdf (accessed 11 September 2007).
6   Wingfield J. The Data Protection Act 1998. *Pharm J* 2000; **265**: 131.
7   Royal Pharmaceutical Society of Great Britain. *Fitness to Practise and Legal Affairs Directorate Fact Sheet: twelve. Confidentiality, the Data Protection Act 1998 and the disclosure of information.* www.rpsgb.org/ pdfs/factsheet12.pdf (accessed 11 September 2007).
8   Royal Pharmaceutical Society of Great Britain. *Medicines, Ethics and*

Practice. A guide for pharmacists and pharmacy technicians. Number 30. London: Royal Pharmaceutical Society of Great Britain, 2006.

9   National Patient Safety Agency. www.npsa.nhs.uk/npsa/about (accessed 11 September 2007).

10   NHS, National Patient Safety Agency. *Root Cause Analysis.* www.npsa. nhs.uk/health/resources/root_cause_analysis (accessed 11 September 2007).

11   Eastham S. Eliminating errors pharmacy update. *Chemist and Druggist* 2002; 29 June: 17–20.

12   News item. Government chooses three routes for evaluating electronic transfer of prescription. *Pharm J* 2001: **266**: 451.

13   Mundy D, Chadwick DW. *The Benefits in and Barriers to the Implementation of the Electronic Transfer of Prescriptions within the United Kingdom National Health Service.* Salford: ISI University of Salford. www.cs.kent.ac.uk/pubs/2003/2073/content.pdf (accessed 11 September 2007).

14   Department of Health. *Statutory Instrument 2004 No 1768 The National Health Service (Complaints) Regulations 2004.* www.opsi.gov.uk/SI/si2004/20041768.htm (accessed 11 September 2007).

15   Pharmaceutical Services Negotiating Committee. *Clinical Governance: Complaints.* www.psnc.org.uk/index.php?type=more_news&id=1576 (accessed 11 September 2007).

16   National Prescribing Centre. *Patient Group Directions. A practical guide and framework of competencies for all professionals using patient group directions.* www.npc.co.uk/publications/pgd/pgd.pdf (accessed 11 September 2007).

17   Department of Health. *Improving Patients' Access to Medicines: a guide to implementing nurse and pharmacist independent prescribing within the NHS in England.* London: Department of Health, 2006. www.dh.gov.uk/PublicationsAndStatistics/Publications/PublicationsPolicyAndGuidance/PublicationsPolicyAndGuidanceArticle/fs/en?CONTENT_ID=4133743&chk=HSzl1/ (accessed 11 September 2007).

18   Pharmaceutical Services Negotiating Committee. *Pharmacist Prescribing. Independent Pharmacist Prescribing. Supplementary Prescribing.* www.psnc.org.uk/index.php?type=page&pid=48&k=5 (accessed 11 September 2007).

19   National Prescribing Centre. *PCT Responsibilities around Prescribing and Medicines Management. A scoping and support guide.* www.npc.co.uk/publications/pctResp/pct_responsibilities.pdf (accessed 11 September 2007).

20   Department of Health. *The NHS Plan: a plan for investment, a plan for reform.* London: Department of Health, 2000.

21   Department of Health. *Building on the Best Choice, Responsiveness and Equity in the NHS.* London: Department of Health, 2003. www.dh.gov.uk/en/Publicationsandstatistics/Publications/PublicationsPolicyAndGuidance/DH_4075302 (accessed 11 September 2007).

8

Responding to symptoms

When people talk, listen completely. Most people never listen.
(Ernest Hemingway)

Checkpoint

Before reading on, think about the following questions to identify
your own knowledge gaps in this area:

- What are some of the problems associated with responding to
  symptoms in a pharmacy?
- What are some of the limitations of using acronyms such as the
  WWHAM method when responding to symptoms?
- How can responding to symptoms in a pharmacy be audited?
- What factors may influence a pharmacist when making a product
  recommendation?

Responding to symptoms has always been an integral part of the pharmacist's role. For many years the general public has utilised this free
service provided by a highly accessible and knowledgeable healthcare
professional. With the introduction of the National Health Service in
1948, all medical treatment and medicines became available to the entire
population free of charge. This provision also included the treatment of
minor ailments and resulted in reduced numbers of people approaching
the pharmacist for advice. It was not until 30 years later that the government realised that NHS costs, particularly the drugs bill, were spiralling
out of control. A related issue was that general practitioners (GPs) were
spending too much of their consultation time on patients with minor ailments, that could be more appropriately screened by other healthcare professionals. To address these concerns the government started to disallow
many over-the-counter (OTC) medicines so that they could no longer be
prescribed on NHS prescriptions. There was also a policy introduced of
reclassifying medicines used for minor ailments from prescription only
medicines (POM) to pharmacy medicines (P), so that they could be purchased in a pharmacy without the need for a prescription.

In 1986 the Nuffield report into the future of pharmacy presented a much wider role for community pharmacists, including more involvement in the treatment of minor ailments.[1] The Royal Pharmaceutical Society of Great Britain (RPSGB) strategy document *Pharmacy in a New Age* further underlined the role of the community pharmacist in managing minor illnesses.[2] The issue of patient self-care was raised higher on the government agenda in 2000 with the publication of the policy document on the future of the NHS, *The NHS Plan*.[3] A policy document *Pharmacy in the Future* was also published in the same year.[4] NHS Direct, the national direct-access telephone service for healthcare was introduced nationally in 2000. One of the aims of this nurse-led service is to provide healthcare advice in response to specific health queries. Since 2002 community pharmacies have been included as an official point of referral from NHS Direct. The issue of self-care was further highlighted in the 2005 government publication *Self-care – a Real Choice: self-care support – a practical option*.[5] With the introduction of the new national contract for pharmacy, 'self-care' was included as an essential service, and the provision of pharmacy-based minor ailment schemes recognised as an enhanced service. The introduction of independent prescribing by pharmacists also offers other possibilities for involvement of pharmacists in responding to symptoms. For example the independent pharmacist prescriber will increase access to medicines for those patients who find the cost of OTC medicines prohibitive and are exempt from prescription charges.

Today it is thought that a community pharmacist practising in an 'average' community pharmacy on a typical day will respond to symptoms presented by between five and fifteen patients. The aim of this chapter is to discuss some of the more practical issues involved in responding to symptoms in a community pharmacy. The main areas to be considered are summarised in Figure 8.1.

There are a number of factors that make responding to symptoms in the pharmacy particularly challenging for the pharmacist:

- there is no access to the patient's medical notes or history
- there are only limited opportunities for a physical examination
- diagnostic testing is not used
- a detailed conversation needs to be initiated
- the customer may have already approached another member of staff
- the issue of privacy may be a concern
- the symptoms may be presented on behalf of another person
- the patient may already have sought advice, information or treatment from another source.

All of these factors need to be considered when a customer approaches the pharmacist and requests advice. In spite of these potential barriers, a

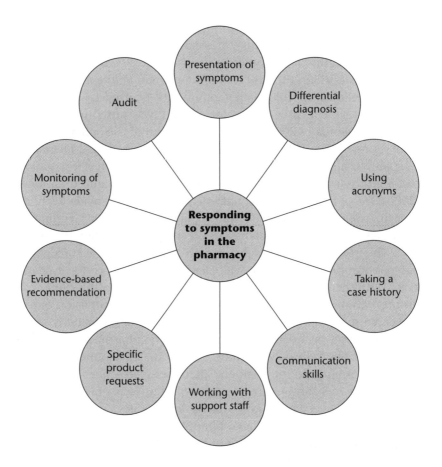

Figure 8.1 Factors to be considered when responding to symptoms in the pharmacy.

positive interaction is possible through excellent communication skills and effective team working with pharmacy support staff.

Presentation of symptoms

The decision to seek professional advice about symptoms is a complex issue. For example there are many differences of public opinion about what symptoms are important and at what point the symptoms should be presented for a professional opinion. For example, surveys have shown that gastrointestinal symptoms such as rectal bleeding, irritable bowel syndrome and dyspepsia are present in 15–40% of the general population, but that only a quarter of this number seek medical advice about them.[6] At the outset, the pharmacist needs to establish who the customer is, as many pharmacy consultations are by proxy, for example parents and grandparents requesting advice on children's conditions, individuals seeking advice on behalf of their partner or someone calling in to the pharmacy for a work colleague over a busy lunchtime. One study identified that pharmacists estimated that one in ten of all consultations were by proxy.[7] It may not be possible to gain all the necessary information if the patient is not present, and in some cases the patient will have to present in the pharmacy for a satisfactory outcome.

It is possible that the person presenting with symptoms has already been referred by another healthcare professional. This is not always obvious at the start of the conversation. Typical case scenarios include:

- a man with a sore-looking red eye requesting something for dry eyes. On closer questioning it emerges that he has already been examined by his optometrist who has advised him to obtain some drops from the pharmacy to moisten the eye
- a catering assistant presents with an itchy hand that looks like a mild form of dermatitis. It is only after considerable questioning that she explains she knows about the condition as she has already been to her GP.

A lot of time and duplicated effort can be saved by asking appropriate questions in the opening stage of the conversation to establish if other healthcare professionals have already been presented with the symptoms.

In some cases the patient contacts the pharmacist by telephone as they may feel more comfortable with this method of communication. Sometimes the phone call is a result of calling NHS Direct. It is not unknown for customers to telephone two or more local pharmacies to compare the advice given in each case. One of the problems with telephone conversations in general is that there is a lack of visual clues and non-verbal feedback. This can lead to a somewhat stilted history taking and a provisional diagnosis before all areas of the problem have been adequately explored. A general principle when taking a telephone history is to try and initially ask the enquirer to state their problem without interruption. It is vital that the same information is collected as with a face-to-face consultation. To avoid misunderstandings it may be necessary to reflect information back to the enquirer to ensure that it has been understood correctly.

Increasingly, pharmacies have their own websites which provide the visitor with the opportunity to contact the pharmacy online. This can lead to all sorts of queries about symptoms and in many cases the information given is brief and inadequate. The RPSGB Code of Ethics has supporting documentation on the professional standards and guidance for internet pharmacy services. When a pharmacy medicine is requested or recommended online, pharmacists must ensure that sufficient information is available to enable a professional assessment of the request and that they provide appropriate counselling and advice. If the patient's symptoms indicate that they would be better served by a face-to-face consultation, they should be advised to consult a pharmacy in person. The identity of the pharmacist assuming professional responsibility for the provision of the advice should be identified on the website.

Making a differential diagnosis

The overall aim of responding to symptoms is to make a clear distinction between a minor illness and a more serious condition that needs to be referred. Typically a pharmacist uses a four-stage process:

- patient assessment based on the obvious information provided by the patient themselves. This leads to a potential provisional diagnosis, usually in the form of a number of options
- questioning the patient to determine specific information that will assist the diagnostic process further and also eliminate more serious conditions
- confirmation, clarification and summary of the available information. At this stage the pharmacist usually asks a few further questions to confirm their provisional diagnosis
- recommendation or outcome of the consultation. This may take the form of offering an OTC medicine and advice or simply offering advice and reassurance. Alternatively it may involve signposting and referral to another healthcare professional.

Although the widely used method of using an acronym is not an ideal vehicle for obtaining information from the patient, the WWHAM acronym is still a popular method used by pharmacy support staff:

W: Who is the patient?
W: What are the symptoms?
H: How long have the symptoms been present?
A: Action taken?
M: Medication being taken?

In practice this acronym provides very little information and it can appear to be very rigid and predictable to be on the receiving end of such questioning.

The WWHAM method provides an overall picture of the presenting complaint but can miss vital information such as the general appearance of the patient, history of any previous symptoms or significant lifestyle or

Table 8.1 Examples of different acronyms used when responding to symptoms in a pharmacy

SIT DOWN SIR		ASMETHOD		ENCORE	
S	Site or location	A	Age/appearance?	E	Explore
I	Intensity or severity	S	Self/someone else?	N	No medication
T	Type or nature	M	Medication?	C	Care
D	Duration	E	Extra medicines?	O	Observe
O	Onset	T	Time persisting	R	Refer
W	With (other symptoms)	H	History?	E	Explain
N	aNnoyed or aggravated by	O	Other symptoms?		
S	Spread or radiation	D	Danger symptoms?		
I	Incidence/frequency pattern				
R	Relieved by				

social factors that may impact on the presenting condition. This acronym may be of some value in the initial screening of a patient by a medicine counter assistant but has limited value in terms of making a differential diagnosis.

Other acronyms that have been developed for use by pharmacists are outlined in Table 8.1. These methods aim to elicit more information but are still considered to be less than ideal as all patients are different and it is unlikely that the acronym can be applied fully to all patients.

Example 8.1   Case study using acronyms

Jason O'Leary is 25 and works as a barman in a local nightclub. He works irregular antisocial hours. He is generally healthy and takes no prescribed medication. During the winter months he gets quite a few colds and blames this on customers coughing and sneezing near him in the nightclub.

This winter he has had two colds in quick succession and each cold seems to start with a sore throat. For the past four days his throat has felt quite sore, especially when he swallows, but he has no other symptoms. He looked in the bathroom mirror this morning and noticed that his throat was looking a little red and inflamed. He decides to go along to the local pharmacy for some advice.

SIT DOWN SIR

S: Site or location – throat
I: Intensity or severity – quite sore
T: Type or nature – worse on swallowing
D: Duration – four days
O: Onset – usually associated with cold
W: With (other symptoms) – no other symptoms
N: annoyed or aggravated by – no information
S: Spread or radiation – no spread of symptoms
I: Incidence or frequency pattern – two recent colds and usually associated with sore throat
R: Relieved by – has not tried any medication, throat continually sore but worse on swallowing

$\rightarrow$

The nature and severity of the problem has been established but there has been no consideration of the appearance of the patient or general lifestyle factors. This method has missed out the fact that the patient's throat looks a little inflamed, that he is generally healthy and the condition is not caused by medication. All of these factors could be significant in the differential diagnosis of a simple acute sore throat.

ASMETHOD

A: Age/appearance? – 25-year-old male, looks generally healthy but a little run down as if he is not taking care of himself
S: Self or someone else? – requesting information for himself
M: Medication? – no regular medication
E: Extra medicines? – has not taken anything for the sore throat
T: Time persisting – 4 days
H: History? – has a tendency to have sore throats associated with cold symptoms, blames this on workplace
O: Other symptoms? – no other symptoms
D: Danger symptoms? – no symptoms to cause concern

In this example there is some exploration of patient history but the exact nature and intensity of the symptoms is not taken into account and any surrounding issues such as social, family or workplace factors are not pursued in any depth.

ENCORE

E: Explore – sore throat symptoms – little information apart from throat looks a little sore
N: No medication – not taking any medication – not an adverse drug reaction
C: Care – No warning symptoms are present – for example bacterial infection such as swollen glands or white tonsil exudate. Sore throat only of 4 days' duration.
O: Observe – 25-year-old male, looks generally healthy but a little run down as if he is not taking care of himself
R: Refer – no need to refer in this case
E: Explain – suck a lozenge or pastille to soothe throat – could select local anaesthetic lozenge or analgesic lozenge – check on suitability; take a systemic painkiller such as paracetamol tablets – explain dose; advise to see GP if the throat is severe/persistent lasting more than 2 weeks or not associated with cold symptoms.

The appearance of the patient is taken into account and any symptoms that would suggest a more serious condition are eliminated. The disadvantage of this method is that the 'refer' and 'explain' sections do not really add to the differential diagnosis.

Taking a case history

Traditionally a pharmacist asks a series of structured questions but does not record a case history. This is in contrast to a GP who takes a formal case history, assesses the symptoms and, if necessary, makes a provisional diagnosis that is later confirmed by further tests or assessment. A typical history-taking format used in medical practice is outlined in Box 8.1.

Box 8.1   Stages involved in taking a patient history[8]

- *Presenting complaint (PC)*: the patient's own account of their condition. The patient is not interrupted but allowed to explain in their own words.
- *History of presenting complaint (HPC)*: when did it start? Have you ever had the condition before? How did you notice the condition? The site and character of the symptoms, any associated features, exacerbating or alleviating factors.
- *Direct questioning (DQ)*: specific questions related to the potential diagnosis.
- *Past medical history (PMH)*: illnesses, operations. For example ask specifically about diabetes, asthma, high blood pressure or epilepsy.
- *Medications/allergies*: prescribed and OTC or herbal medicines.
- *Social/family history (SH/FH)*: brief exploration of any relevant social or family history.
- *Functional enquiry*: this aims to uncover undeclared symptoms by further questioning to determine factors such as recent weight loss, fatigue, fevers and recent trauma.

The history-taking approach assumes a more formal face-to-face, uninterrupted clinical environment which is not the norm in a community pharmacy. It is precisely the informal and accessible nature of the pharmacy that patients see as a benefit to requesting advice on symptoms. A compromise is therefore needed to guard against the rigid use of limited acronyms and the more detailed history taking that would be impractical in a community pharmacy setting. The challenge for the pharmacist is to obtain meaningful information in a flexible and yet structured way.

Communication skills in the pharmacy

International research into the needs of patients when they receive counselling in a pharmacy can be summarised by the following statements.[9]

The patient wants:

- to feel confident in the quality of the counselling
- a high-quality interaction
- to feel privacy is respected
- to feel there is a genuine concern
- a friendly and relaxed atmosphere
- reassurance about their problem
- to be given reasons for the pharmacist asking questions
- sufficient information.

Confidence in the quality of the counselling and the interaction will depend on the pharmacist taking sufficient time to gain important information before offering advice. A rushed consultation where the pharmacist appears distracted or gives the impression that they have been interrupted will not put a patient at their ease. The patient must be allowed to state their case clearly and be able to engage fully in the interaction. The quality of interaction can sometimes be influenced by the first impressions that are made. For example the appearance of the pharmacist, their demeanour and tone of speech will all influence the way the consultation proceeds. Conversely, the pharmacist may be influenced by how the patient presents their case, their appearance, age, sex or if they appear to be particularly demanding or aggressive. In theory a truly professional approach would not be hindered by any of these variables. In practice anecdotal evidence suggests that these factors all have a real impact on how the counselling proceeds. A key activity to overcoming any prejudice on the initial contact is to listen carefully to the enquirer. This involves important but too often neglected listening skills such as:

- paying full attention to the patient and avoiding any distractions
- using appropriate body language to show that the patient has your attention
- making an effort to see if there is any hidden meaning in the statements that are being made. For example the symptoms may be played down. The statement 'It is only a headache' may be taken at face value or it may be more significant depending on the tone of voice used
- taking the time to reflect back to the patient to clarify what has been said.

The issue of privacy in the pharmacy has already been discussed and this sensitive area needs to be resolved at an early stage in the consultation. This may mean that the customer is happy to discuss their symptoms in the medicine counter area or would prefer to use a private consultation room. Some customers prefer a compromise between these two extremes and would prefer the conversation to take place in a quieter area of the pharmacy, but not in a designated consultation area. This involves the pharmacist interpreting verbal or non-verbal signals and possibly moving away from the medicine counter for a more private conversation. Some customers may be drawn to the informal retail setting of a community pharmacy and can feel threatened by the clinical atmosphere of a consultation room. The pharmacist has to make a rapid assessment of the level of privacy that the customer is looking for. This will depend on a number of factors such as the nature of the symptoms and the customers' individual preferences and expectations.

For the customer to feel there is a genuine concern, the pharmacist needs an empathetic approach. To develop this approach requires considerable self-discipline and a clear recognition that the community pharmacist is generally dealing with people who are either unwell or are offering care and support for a family member or friend. There should be the recognition that illness brings with it differing amounts of uncertainty, stress, fear and dependency. It is only by making an attempt to view a problem from the other person's perspective that a positive outcome can be achieved.

A friendly, relaxed atmosphere can sometimes be difficult to generate in a busy dispensing environment. The pharmacist has an influential role in terms of the ethos of an individual pharmacy. Other staff members are guided by the way in which a pharmacist interacts with different customers. Using a professional approach, it is not always straightforward to strike the correct balance between friendliness and making the consultation too conversational. For example it is important that the pharmacist is aware of the appropriate point to close the consultation and the customer feels that their concern has been given due consideration. In practice this can be quite difficult with a particularly talkative customer. Sufficient consideration needs to be given to how to keep the conversation professional and yet open and friendly. Reassurance about a problem is sometimes the main outcome when responding to symptoms. If the presenting symptoms do not warrant referral to another healthcare professional and no medication is needed, it is vital that the reassurance is communicated in a positive way so that the patient does not feel shortchanged. It is also important to avoid any false reassurance if there is an element of uncertainty or the symptoms need to be investigated further. The outcome needs to be left open but with the strong advice that the symptoms will need further investigation from their GP.

Questioning is an important skill, and from the customer's perspective the questions are more acceptable if a reason is given for asking questions. Before proceeding with a series of seemingly unrelated questions it is useful to put the conversation into context (Example 8.2).

As a decision is reached about the presenting symptoms the customer expects to be given a certain amount of information. The provision

---

Example 8.2   Customer presenting with indigestion symptoms

Pharmacist: 'To find out a little more about your indigestion I need to ask a few questions.'

The pharmacist then proceeds with the established 'funnel approach' where the first questions are open questions to encourage the customer to start providing information and then using more closed questions to narrow down the detail.

Pharmacist: 'How would you describe your indigestion?' (open question)
Customer: 'It's like a burning feeling in my stomach after I've eaten. I sometimes feel a bit sick and get acid in my throat.'
Pharmacist: 'How long have you noticed these symptoms for?' (closed question)
Customer: 'A few days ago I went out for a curry and since then I seem to have been very unsettled.'

The pharmacist is starting to come closer to a differential diagnosis but is more likely to gain co-operation if the reason behind the questioning is stated at the outset.

---

of sufficient information in terms of how to use the recommended product, lifestyle advice, preventative measures and information on the condition all add value to the pharmacist–customer interaction. The depth and quantity of information is often dictated by the nature of the symptoms. For example an anxious parent wanting information on headlice treatment or acne products is likely to require a considerable amount of information. By contrast, a customer may have a specific question about a condition or product and appear to be in a rush. Well-developed listening skills are needed to gauge the most appropriate level of information required. Communication skills such as well-developed empathy, questioning and listening are essential attributes in this area of pharmacy practice.

Effective use of support staff

The medicine counter assistant and other members of the pharmacy support team have a prominent frontline role in responding to symptoms in the pharmacy. Provided that the customer does not specifically request to speak to a pharmacist, or the symptoms or condition presented are not identified on the medicine sales protocol as referral symptoms, it is unlikely that the customer will speak to a pharmacist. In one study counter assistants managed 84% of all requests for deregulated medicines without any involvement or input from the pharmacist.[10] The use of support staff in this way is dependent on the use of a medicines protocol and a minimum standard of staff training as discussed in Chapter 3.

For the pharmacist to manage their time effectively they are reliant on the skills and knowledge of others and their capacity to adhere to agreed protocols. As the healthcare professional with responsibility for providing this service, the pharmacist must ensure that this largely delegated task is of the highest standard. An example of good practice is outlined in the case study 8.1.

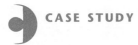 CASE STUDY

Case study 8.1

A customer approaches Jane who is an experienced counter assistant and asks her for some antibiotic drops for sore red eyes. Jane checks that the customer is happy to answer a few questions to see if this is the most suitable product for her. The customer looks a little dubious as she is in a rush but the soreness of her eyes is becoming a constant irritation so she decides to co-operate. Jane proceeds to ask a number of open questions to establish the nature of the symptoms. A few more closed questions are used to narrow down the differential diagnosis. During the course of the conversation the customer mentions that they take some regular tablets which they obtain on a prescription. The customer cannot remember the name of the medication but confirms that they have had their prescription medication dispensed from your pharmacy. Before proceeding with the consultation further Jane asks the patient if they are happy for a few notes to be taken and shown to the pharmacist. Jane notes down the main details of the consultation and also checks the patient medication record (PMR) to find the patient details. A minute later Jane approaches the pharmacist who has just finished a telephone conversation. The pharmacist reads the following that has been jotted down in a notepad:

→

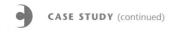

CASE STUDY (continued)

- sore red eyes – described as dry for past 3 months
- no discharge, very uncomfortable but not painful
- given up wearing contact lenses a month ago, rubs eyes a lot as they feel irritated
- PMR: Prempak C

The pharmacist finds the efficient and professional approach of Jane very reassuring for a number of reasons:

- customers are dealt with in a polite and considerate manner and their requests are treated in a logical and systematic way
- the agreed protocol for different conditions is always adhered to
- the assistant has a clear idea of where the boundary of her responsibility lies and always works within established guidelines
- the written and highlighted information summary avoids unnecessary repetition when the pharmacist is asked to intervene in the consultation
- the pharmacist's time is saved by the assistant accessing the PMR and finding out any additional background information
- the assistant is discreet in their approach.

Some of the more common problems encountered when support staff are delegated to deal with responding to symptoms are:

- there is no clear explanation to the customer of the need to ask questions and why this approach is being used
- the consultation proceeds too far before the pharmacist is involved
- information provided by the customer that is sometimes of a sensitive nature is repeated in front of the customer to the pharmacist
- inadequate information is obtained from the customer and a sale of a product is agreed with very little dialogue or interaction
- the assistant lacks confidence and involves the pharmacist unnecessarily without asking some preliminary questions. Conversely the assistant is over-confident and has a tendency to offer wrong information that is not evidence based
- the assistant does not explain clearly to the pharmacist all of the relevant details of the case so that the pharmacist has to retrace the original conversation, which can be inconvenient and puzzling for the customer
- the medicines protocol is not adhered to and the assistant deviates from the agreed guidelines.

The quality of the customer experience is totally dependent on a disciplined and logical approach to information gathering, within a flexible conversational framework. The ongoing training and development of the pharmacy team in this area is a key priority for any community pharmacist.

Specific product requests

Some customers prefer to ask for a specific product by name rather than ask openly for advice about a condition. This type of purchasing behaviour can be due to a number of factors:

- from past experience the customer has found a particular product successful in treating a recurrent condition and is aware of the signs and symptoms
- the customer has taken advice from family or friends
- the influence of heavy advertising on branded products.

There is evidence that this type of customer may become puzzled or hostile if questioned about their choice of purchase. Pharmacy staff may feel uncomfortable about interacting with this type of purchaser.[11] The phenomenon of the 'determined purchaser' is well established as a type of customer behaviour in community pharmacy. When responding to a specific product request it is important to establish if the purchaser has used the product before. The way in which any questions are asked will influence the outcome of the interaction with the customer.

Powerful consumer advertising of recently deregulated medicines from POM to P can certainly cause problems. For example the deregulation of chloramphenicol eye drops resulted in consumers wishing to purchase this product for a number of indications outside the product licence. This was mainly in response to advertising and requires considerable sensitivity and tact to explain that the purchase would not be appropriate. This potentially difficult area emphasises the need to frame all questions carefully and to give some indication to the purchaser why questions are being asked.

Evidence-based recommendations

The public is entitled to expect that medicines purchased over the counter will be safe, effective and appropriate for the condition to be treated.

The profession expects pharmacists to ensure that they are

competent in any area in which such advice is given to the public.[12] As part of ongoing continuing professional development the pharmacist may need to spend some time reflecting on the advice provided and comparing their advice with the most recent evidence. It is sometimes possible to become complacent about which products are recommended without referring to evidence-based guidelines. Recommendations can be influenced by factors such as:

- a 'favourite', well-established product that has been recommended for years and forms part of an ingrained behavioural response to a particular condition
- a judgemental approach to the customer in terms of offering a product that would be an acceptable price
- the range of products on the medicines counter and the way that the products are merchandised
- the customer may have an underlying preference throughout the consultation and reject the advice given.

These barriers can sometimes make an evidence-based approach to product recommendation a difficult objective to achieve. A useful approach is to review a specific product category, categorise the products available and examine the evidence base for each product type. This type of activity can lead to a rationalisation of the medicine counter and also involve the pharmacy support team in additional training.

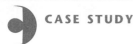

CASE STUDY

Case study 8.2

Alison is a pharmacist working in a pharmacy with high OTC sales. She has noticed an increase in the sales of ear wax-softening products and decides to investigate this product category. The full-time medicine counter assistant tells Alison that her impression is that quite a few older people request this type of product by specific brand name. She says that when recommending a product it can be quite difficult as her understanding is that all of these products are fairly similar. At one time the local practice nurse seemed to routinely syringe ears and now this procedure seems to be quite uncommon. Alison's counter assistant thinks that this may be a reason why sales of these products have increased.

As part of her investigation Alison makes the following notes:

continued overleaf

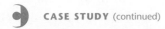

Availability of over-the-counter products for ear wax and evidence-based recommendation

- Cerumenolytics are well-established products to help soften and dislodge impacted ear wax.
- *BNF* [*British National Formulary*] suggests olive and almond oils and sodium bicarbonate as safe.
- Little clinical trial data on the comparison of different products.
- Prodigy website summary[13]: a recent Cochrane systematic review of trials of cerumenolytics found eight clinical trials, all with small numbers of participants, and most of poor methodological quality. The reviewers concluded that there is no evidence to prefer one particular cerumenolytic to any other, and that water and sodium chloride 0.9% seem to be as effective as any proprietary agent. There is the recommendation to use tap water, sodium chloride 0.9% or sodium bicarbonate ear drops. Olive oil and almond oil are widely used and are therefore also included in the choice of products.
- Some evidence that peroxide-based treatments are an effective treatment.[14]
- Very few practical issues as they are very safe products and can be used by all ages and patient groups – they do not interact with other medicines.
- Side-effects very unusual – mainly local irritation or hypersensitivity reactions
- If an OTC product for ear wax has been used correctly and the treatment has failed then the patient should be referred.
- Discussed ear syringing with practice nurse, and the medical centre has reduced this procedure as softening with ear drops is the preferred method of treatment.

As a result of this investigation Alison decides to draft a new protocol for the sale of cerumenolytics and hold a briefing meeting for members of the pharmacy team. By reviewing the evidence base a number of other issues are raised about the quality of advice given when supplying these products.

Complementary medicines

The Royal Pharmaceutical Society of Great Britain (RPSGB) supporting documentation on the sale and supply of medicines states that the pharmacist must assist patients to make informed decisions by providing them with necessary and relevant information when supplying complementary therapies.[12]

With a high public interest in complementary therapies there is an increasing demand for the pharmacist to become involved in this area. This means that there is increasing pressure for the pharmacist to express a view on specific complementary products.

Monitoring of symptoms

The vast majority of symptoms that are treated in the pharmacy are self-limiting and it is anticipated that the treatment will last only a short time period or the condition will be referred. One of the disadvantages of the consultation in the pharmacy is that the pharmacist does not obtain feedback on the outcome of the treatment. Sometimes a customer will offer feedback that is either positive or negative on their next visit to the pharmacy. This can sometimes be a long time after the event and the interaction with the customer can seem like a distant memory. In some cases where it is deemed to be of clinical significance a record is made of an OTC sale in the PMR. Routine record keeping of all consultations and OTC sales is not currently standard practice as this would be both onerous and have a negative impact on the speedy access to informal consultation and advice.

In some cases it is useful to encourage the patient to contact the pharmacy to inform the pharmacist of the outcome of their symptoms or how they have responded to using a particular product. This can have benefits for both the pharmacist in terms of an informal self-audit of their service and also the customer in improving the ongoing level of support provided. It is sometimes appropriate to use a simple statement such as: 'Let me know how you get on with this product' or 'Please telephone if your symptoms change or do not improve within two days'.

Examples of when monitoring of symptoms may be appropriate and the customer is encouraged to inform the pharmacist of the outcome or progression of their symptoms are listed below:

- a newly marketed OTC product or a recent POM to P medicine is recommended
- the customer experiences an adverse reaction to the recommended product. The pharmacist will need to document this and ensure that any adverse reaction is reported
- there is a change in the presenting symptoms and the customer would like more information or advice or it may be necessary to refer to their GP.

Audit – responding to symptoms

The process of audit has already been discussed in Chapter 4. The RPSGB website provides a template for an audit of responding to symptoms.[15] The standard is based on the suitability of questioning when a customer presents with a set of symptoms. The aim of the audit is to determine the percentage of customers who are suitably questioned when a specific symptom is presented. To be able to collect meaningful data a fairly common symptom that can be treated with an OTC product needs to be selected. This type of audit is quite time consuming as it involves observational studies and building up data over a defined period of time.

A different approach to audit is to use agreed model standards and a scoring system for each standard. Documentation produced by the Department of Pharmacy Policy and Practice at Keele University provides a means of self-audit and measuring the performance of the pharmacy.[16] Criteria for responding to symptoms include:

- a policy exists to ensure that accurate advice is given to patients by the most appropriate person
- an information system exists to ensure the consistency, safety and appropriateness of recommended products
- a pharmacy staff training policy ensures that customers and patients receive accurate, appropriate and current information.

The set of standards is checked by the auditor to gain a snapshot picture of how the pharmacy is performing in this area.

Responding to symptoms continues to be a key role and an essential service of the community pharmacist. Ongoing CPD in this area is vital for the pharmacist to be able to offer a customer-focused and evidence-based service.

Implications for practice

Activity 1

- Select a suitable OTC category and conduct an observational audit of responding to symptoms in your pharmacy. Decide how you will collect, analyse and use the data.

Activity 2

What are the training needs of your pharmacy team when responding to symptoms?

- Are there common areas that can be identified as a specific training need?
- Are there some specific examples of good practice that can be shared with the wider team?

Directions for question 1: each of the questions or incomplete statements in this section is followed by five suggested answers. Select the best answer in each case.

Q1   If the ASMETHOD mnemonic is used when responding to symptoms, the 'S' is used to denote:

A   Site or location
B   Self or someone else
C   Spread or radiation
D   Symptoms
E   Self-treatment already used

Directions for questions 2 to 3: for each numbered question select the one lettered option above it which is most closely related to it. Within each group of questions each lettered option may be used once, more than once, or not at all.

This question refers to taking a patient history.

A   PC
B   HPC
C   DQ
D   PMH
E   SH/FH

Select from A to E which one of the above fits the following statements:

Q2   A patient presenting with a sore on their foot explains that they have a history of diabetes.
Q3   A patient describes how pain in their sinuses has resulted from a heavy cold that started 2 weeks ago. The patient explains that they have a tendency to suffer from inflammation of the sinuses every winter.

Directions for questions 4 to 8: each of the questions or incomplete statements in this section is followed by three responses. For each question ONE or MORE of the responses is (are) correct. Decide which of the responses is (are) correct. Then choose:

A   if **1**, **2** and **3** are correct
B   if **1** and **2** only are correct
C   if **2** and **3** only are correct
D   if **1** only is correct
E   if **3** only is correct

Directions summarised:
A: 1, 2, 3   B: 1, 2 only   C: 2, 3 only   D: 1 only   E: 3 only

Q4   According to research, a patient requires the following when they receive counselling in a pharmacy:

1   To feel privacy is respected
2   To be given reasons for the pharmacist asking questions
3   A friendly and relaxed atmosphere

Q5   Which of the following are closed questions?

1   How would you describe your cough?
2   Is your cough worse at night?
3   How long have you noticed the symptoms for?

Q6   Making a differential diagnosis involves:

1   Patient assessment to make a provisional diagnosis
2   Questioning to eliminate more serious conditions
3   Taking a detailed medication history

Q7   The use of acronyms such as WWHAM by pharmacy support staff have the following advantages:

1   They provide a lot of information
2   They can help to make a more fluid interaction with the customer
3   They can provide an overall picture of the presenting complaint

Q8   Monitoring of symptoms in the pharmacy may be useful when:

1   Any product is recommended that has been deregulated from POM to P
2   A newly marketed OTC product is recommended
3   The customer experiences an adverse reaction to the recommended product.

Directions for questions 9 and 10: The following questions consist of a statement in the left-hand column followed by a second statement in the right-hand column.
Decide whether the first statement is true or false.

Decide whether the second statement is true or false.
Then choose:

A   if both statements are true and the second statement is a correct
        explanation of the first statement
B   if both statements are true but the second statement is NOT a correct
        explanation of the first statement
C   if the first statement is true but the second statement is false
D   if the first statement is false but the second statement is true
E   if both statements are false

Directions summarised:

A:	True	True	second statement is **a correct explanation** of the first
B:	True	True	second statement is **NOT a correct explanation** of the first
C:	True	False	
D:	False	True	
E:	False	False	

Q9   A young woman asks to purchase some choloramphenicol eye drops as
          her eyes feel dry and sore. On further questioning the pharmacist
          discovers that the dryness is possibly due to the air conditioning in the
          office and a lot of her work involves using a computer screen. After further
          discussion the pharmacist decides to offer an alternative product but the
          customer is insistent on their choice of product. The pharmacist decides to
          supply the chloramphenicol eye drops.

■   *Statement 1*: In this situation this is the correct course of action for the
     pharmacist.
■   *Statement 2*: Heavy consumer advertising of recently deregulated POM
     to P products can lead to the phenomenon of the determined
     purchaser.

Q10   A pharmacist decides to increase the range of herbal medicinal products
          available in their pharmacy.

■   *Statement 1*: The professional responsibility of the pharmacist is to
     ensure that the products are obtained from a reputable source of supply.
■   *Statement 2*: The professional responsibility of the pharmacist is to
     ensure that there is no reason to doubt the quality or safety of the
     products.

Case studies

Level 1

Mark Dean is 19 and is keen on keeping fit. He goes running regularly with a running club and plays squash once a week. His girlfriend

regularly complains that his trainers smell revolting. Mark admits that his feet tend to get quite sweaty and smelly but he always has a shower at the sports centre after each training session.

Over the past week he has noticed that it itches between his toes, especially next to his little toe, and the skin between his toes appears white and soggy. The condition seems to be getting worse and his feet are beginning to feel sore. He decides to go along to the local pharmacy for some advice.

- How do you recognise the clinical features of athlete's foot?
- What questions would you ask Mark Dean to ensure that this condition does not require referral?
- Critically discuss the availability of OTC products for athlete's foot and make an evidence-based recommendation for this patient.

Level 2

Yunus is a preregistration trainee who is working in a large community pharmacy with a busy medicine counter. There is a wide mix of staff working on the medicine counter, ranging from full-time experienced assistants to part-time evening staff. Yunus's tutor has expressed a concern that paracetamol products are being supplied without appropriate questioning and information. He is keen to investigate the extent of this problem and asks Yunus to design an audit on the sale of paracetamol products in the pharmacy.

- What are the benchmark standards that Yunus could select when designing this audit?
- How could the audit be designed?
- What are some of the practical problems and limitations of this type of audit?

Level 3

Colin is pharmacy manager of the community pharmacy of a small multiple. He has become increasingly concerned about Laura who works part-time on the medicines counter. Laura is an experienced counter assistant that has worked in a community pharmacy for a number of years. She is always friendly and helpful with customers. Today Colin was near the medicines counter counselling a customer when he noticed that Laura was approached by a young mother with her baby. Part of the conversation between Laura and the customer is reproduced below:

Customer: 'Do you have anything for colic?'

Laura: 'Oh hello – yes we've got quite a few colic products, let me show you.'

Customer: 'I've heard that they grow out of colic, is that right? It's driving me crazy at the moment.'

Laura: 'They do grow out of it. Have you tried increasing the amount of feed?'

Customer: 'Well, I've made the feeds a bit stronger but it doesn't seem to be working.'

Laura: 'How old is he?'

Customer: '11 weeks and he has spent the past 3 weeks screaming.'

Laura: 'I had the same problem with my first and started her on solids early. I'd recommend going on to solids, you can always try some colic drops as well.'

Customer: 'I suppose I could give it a go.'

- Highlight Colin's concerns about this incident.
- How should Colin approach Laura with these concerns?

References

1   Nuffield Foundation. *A Report to the Nuffield Foundation*. London: Nuffield Foundation, 1986.

2   Royal Pharmaceutical Society of Great Britain. *Pharmacy in a New Age*. London: Royal Pharmaceutical Society of Great Britain, 1995.

3   Department of Health. *The NHS Plan: a plan for investment, a plan for reform*. London. The Stationery Office, 2000.

4   Department of Health. *Pharmacy in the Future. Implementing the NHS Plan*. London: The Stationery Office, 2000.

5   Department of Health. *Self Care – a Real Choice: self care support – a practical option*. London: The Stationery Office, 2005.

6   Jones R. Editorial. Self care. *BMJ* 2000; **320**: 596.

7   Weiss MC, Cantrill JA, Nguyen LY. Pharmacists' and preregistration pharmacy graduates views of proxy consultations. *Int J Pharm Pract* 1998; **6**: 1206.

8   Hope RA, Longmore JM, Wilkinson I, Turok E. *Oxford Handbook of Clinical Medicine*, 5th edn. Oxford: Oxford University Press, 2001.

9   Lumb J. September issue of IJPP: research into patient counselling. *Pharm J* 2003; **271**: 303. www.pjonline.com/Editorial/20030906/articles/ijpp.html (accessed 12 September 2007).

10 Ward PR, Bissell P, Noyce PR. Medicines counter assistants; role and responsibilities in the sale of deregulated medicines. *Int J Pharm Pract* 1998; **6**: 207–215.

11 Morris C, Cantrill J, Weiss M. 'One simple question should be enough': consumers' perceptions of pharmacy protocols. *Int J Pharm Pract* 1997; **5**: 64–71.

12 Royal Pharmaceutical Society of Great Britain. *Professional Standards and Guidance for the Sale and Supply of Medicines, 2007, Standard 8,*

Complementary Therapies and Medicines. London: Royal Pharmaceutical Society of Great Britain, 2007.

13   Prodigy. *Clinical Topic: earwax*. www.prodigy.nhs.uk/earwax/view_whole_guidance (accessed 12 September 2007).

14   Fahmy S, Whitefield M. Multicentre clinical trial of Exterol as a cerumenolytic. *Br J Clin Pract* 1982; **36**: 197–204.

15   Royal Pharmaceutical Society of Great Britain. *Responding to Symptoms*. www.rpsgb.org/pdfs/respond.pdf (accessed 18 September 2007).

16   Department of Pharmacy Policy and Practice Keele University. *Model Standards for Self Audit in Community Pharmacy in England (9) response to symptoms*. www.rpsgb.org/pdfs/chap9.pdf (accessed 18 September 2007).

9

Multidisciplinary working

None of us is as smart as all of us.

(Japanese proverb)

Checkpoint

Before reading on, think about the following questions to identify your own knowledge gaps in this area:

- Why is the improvement of medicines management an urgent priority for the NHS?
- What are the stages involved in setting up a medicines-management service?
- How can a community pharmacist contribute to a hospital discharge scheme?
- How can a community pharmacist work more closely with general practitioners (GPs)?

As experts on medication, community pharmacists have a lot to offer in contributing to the targets of the NHS. To fulfil this potential the pharmacist needs to be fully integrated into the healthcare team and work as part of a multidisciplinary team. The document *A Vision for Pharmacy in the New NHS*[1] identifies ten key roles that will determine the future direction of pharmacy services. Three of the key roles that are especially relevant to team working are listed below:

- to provide medicines-management services, especially for people with enduring illness
- to contribute to seamless and safe medicines management throughout the patient journey
- to support patients as partners in medicine taking.

This chapter includes a review of pharmacist involvement in:

- medicines management and prescribing projects with local GPs
- hospital discharge schemes
- the National Service Frameworks (NSFs) for Older People, Coronary Heart Disease and Diabetes

Successful multidisciplinary working involves being able to present the

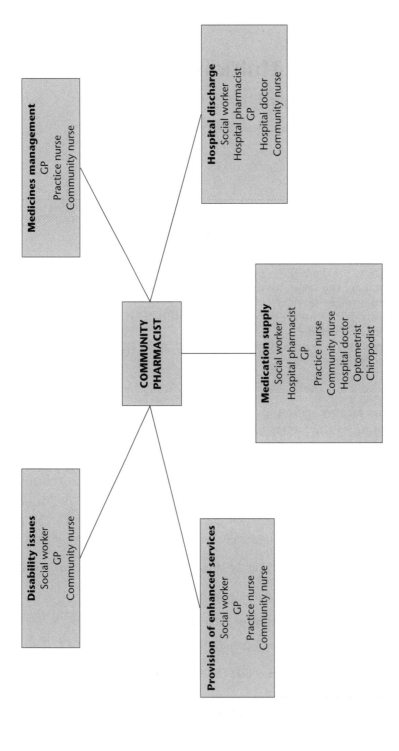

Figure 9.1 Overview of the interaction of the community pharmacist with other professions.

value of pharmacy-based services in a positive way. Sections on negotiation skills and how to make a successful business case for a new service are also included in this chapter. An overview of the interaction of the community pharmacist with other health and social care professions is outlined in Figure 9.1.

Relationships with general practice

Historically, the pharmacist has only contacted the GP when there has been a potential problem with a prescription. This brief interaction is often rushed and at a time when both pharmacist and doctor are under pressure, dealing directly with patients. It is unfortunate that in some cases this has led to a negative relationship between the professions. The agenda of both the pharmacist and the doctor has been brought closer together and is no longer restricted to the confines of this narrow communication. The general medical services (GMS) contract, introduced in 2004, aims to reward GPs who meet targets for providing services. Practice payments are determined by meeting targets that are included in a *Quality and Outcomes Framework* (QOF), which is an evidence-based list of performance indicators for a number of clinical areas. There is the expectation that GPs will develop new working relationships with other healthcare professionals to help them meet their contractual targets. Pharmacists are ideally placed to form working partnerships. However, there is still considerable misunderstanding about the potential broader role of the pharmacist, which may stem from a suspicion of their retail background.

In response to the All-party Pharmacy Group Inquiry into the Future of Pharmacy, the Royal Pharmaceutical Society of Great Britain (RPSGB) stated that there must be a concerted effort to create links between the pharmacy and GP contracts.[2] Collaboration between doctors and pharmacists is needed to meet the government's aspirations for supporting patients with long-term conditions, and will involve the sharing of patient information.[3]

Medicines management

Over 700 million prescription items are dispensed in England each year at a total cost approaching £8billion.[4] There is strong evidence to suggest that help is needed to enable people to make the best use of their medicines. For example, there are compliance problems with up to half of all medicines prescribed, and up to 17% of hospital admissions are related to problems with medication. Medicines management is a term that has several definitions, the simplest of which is 'enabling people to make the best possible use of medicines'. The National Prescribing Centre website has a number of useful resources to assist individuals and organisations to make improvements in medicines management.[5]

Medicines management is not the same as the advanced service, medicines use review. It is an enhanced service similar to a Level 3 medication review where there is face-to-face contact with the patient and access to the patient's notes. However medicines management is more than a medication review as it offers a more patient-centred approach that involves a discussion of the patient's lifestyle as well as the medication regimen. For a medicines-management programme to work there must be a good relationship between the pharmacist, the patient and the GP.

Improving medicines management is an urgent priority for the NHS. Both the GMS contract and the contractual framework for community pharmacists refer to medicines management and many of the NSFs include medicines management as a key development area.

Collaborative involvement in medicines-management projects will require a certain amount of resource in terms of time and additional cost. However, improved medicines management will help free up resources that can be put to better use. Examples of the positive benefits of medicines management include:

- a more efficient repeat-prescribing system may release time for longer and more meaningful GP consultations and reduce administrative workload
- a review of residential home ordering procedures may help prevent community pharmacies having to redispense items unnecessarily
- a timely medication review may prevent a patient's admission to hospital.

The Community Pharmacy Medicines Management Project (CPMMP) is a research project to evaluate the medicines management by community pharmacists for patients with a confirmed diagnosis of coronary heart disease.[6] The specific definition of medicines management in this project was an intervention between the pharmacist, patient and GP. The aim of the intervention process was to:

- deliver measurable health gain to the patient
- deliver improvements to value for money in medicines prescribing, and cost reductions for the NHS
- construct a new approach to patient care by extending the partnership between pharmacist, patient and physician

- facilitate collaboration between the health professionals in primary care
- maximise the use of the skills and training of the community pharmacist.

The project involved 1493 patients, 50 pharmacies, 62 pharmacists and 39 GP practices. The main findings from the project were that:

- the GPs in the study were generally supportive of working more closely with their pharmacist colleagues. Sometimes concerns were expressed about professional boundaries and responsibilities and the potential for the duplication of effort and there were some issues with accessing confidential patient information
- practice staff were also supportive of working more closely with pharmacists.

Stages in setting up a medicines-management service

A medicines-management resource pack for community pharmacists, available from the www.medicinesmanagement.org.uk website, provides useful information for pharmacists interested in delivering a medicines-management service in a community pharmacy setting.[7] To help community pharmacists to become involved in a local medicines-management project there are ten suggested stages. These stages are summarised in Figure 9.2.

Identify local need

The first stage involves working with the local primary care trust (PCT) to identify health needs in the area, talking to local GP practices to find out their priorities in the GMS QOF.

Assess suitability of premises

A consultation area is necessary to deliver a medicines-management service as the consultation needs to be uninterrupted. This facility may already be in place for providing medicines use reviews (MURs).

Assess individual skill and knowledge – CPD

Apply the continuing professional development (CPD) cycle to identify any learning needs and plan how these needs can be met (Ch. 1). This will be specific for the project and individual pharmacist. This process should include a self-assessment of both clinical knowledge and communication skills. If a list of generic competencies is available this can act

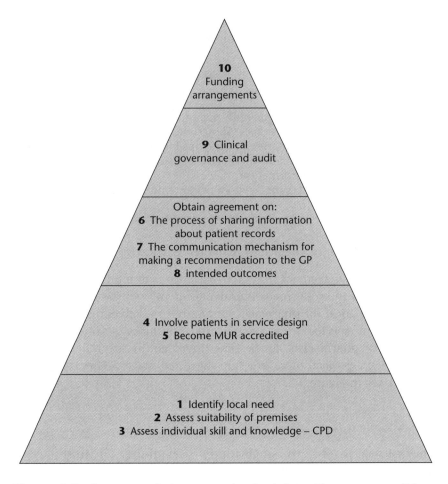

Figure 9.2 Summary of the stages involved in setting up a medicines-management service. CPD, continuing professional development; GP, general practitioner; MUR, medicines use review.

as a useful starting point for identifying learning needs. Development of members of the support team will also need to be considered.

Involve patients in service design

Speak informally to a number of patients about a proposed medicines-management service to ascertain their views on what they would expect from the service, how long they would expect a consultation to last and what they would expect to gain from the service. Use these comments to provide a selection of patients with an outline of the proposed service, and ask for their feedback.

Become MUR accredited

Experience of offering an MUR service can be seen as a useful developmental step in offering a full medicines-management service. Further information on how to become accredited to offer this service is provided in Chapter 5.

Obtain agreement on the process of sharing information about patient records

The Caldicott Report on the review of patient-identifiable information outlines principles of good practice relating to the use of patient-identifiable information within the NHS.[8] The report makes provision for the exchange of information between healthcare professionals in appropriate circumstances.

The proposed medicines-management project, confidentiality of patient information and any issues of patient confidentiality must be discussed with the PCT Caldicott guardian. Areas to be agreed on include how information will be stored and the arrangements in place for informing patients of the processes involved.

Obtain agreement on the communication mechanism for making a recommendation to the GP

Arrangements for the communication of information and recommendations to the patient's GP need to be agreed with the local practice. In many cases this may include devising and piloting a standard electronic form and checking that it fulfils the requirements of both pharmacist and GP. A closed loop system to confirm that information has been received by the GP and which recommendations have been implemented needs to be tested.

Obtain agreement on intended outcomes

Identify with the commissioners of the service (PCT and/or GP) how the service will be assessed by agreeing what outcomes will be measured. The outcomes should be easy to measure, such as: number of patients seen, medication changed and related to the GMS QOF.

Clinical governance and audit

Discuss how the quality of the proposed service will be measured and what aspects of the service will be selected for audit and assessment.

Funding arrangements

Agree funding arrangements either as an enhanced service within the pharmacy contract or as a local practice-based commissioning arrangement.

Funding arrangements may well be a barrier to launching the service and this is discussed further in the next section on making a business case for a new service.

Making a business case for a new service

When making a business case for a new service it is essential to view the service from the point of view of the primary care organisation (PCO). It is useful to ask such questions as:

- does the service solve a PCO problem?
- does the service meet an unmet patient or PCO need?
- does the service add value to or complement an existing service?
- does the service help to meet PCO targets such as reduced waiting times in primary care?

The type of service selected will depend on the gaps in the current service provision. There are three main routes for establishing a new service:

- if the pharmacist is in good communication with local GP practices, this can lead to informal discussion and ideas for new services
- the GMS contract and NSFs set out the specific targets that PCOs have to meet and this can be a useful starting point when in the initial stages of selecting a service
- examine strategic documents published by the PCO that may indicate possible gaps in current service provision.

A formal bid for a new service should be set out as a standardised document.[9] Using minor ailments as an example, the type of information required in each section of the document is summarised in Table 9.1.

Top tips for preparing a bid

- Discuss your provisional ideas with local stakeholders.
- Seek advice from colleagues who have provided a similar service.
- Find out the priorities of your local PCO.
- Be able to demonstrate your competence to deliver the service.
- Develop any necessary protocols.
- Search for evidence of the proposed positive benefits of the service.
- Design ways of monitoring service quality and demonstrating effectiveness.

Table 9.1 Preparation of a formal bid for a new service

Document section	*Suggested contents*
Title	The title page gives a clear indication of the type of proposed service. Example: minor ailments service.
Executive summary	This section of the document establishes the need for the service and the evidence base. It would be useful to include information on the level of deprivation in the local area, percentage of GP time spent on local ailments and the impact on offering an improved and accessible primary healthcare service. In view of the limited PCO resources and PCO accountability for spending money, the evidence base for any new proposal needs to be clearly summarised.[9]
Background and introduction	The background and introduction to the proposal is a detailed referenced overview of why the service is important at a local level and the specific need that it fulfils.
Proposal	The details of the proposal explain how the service will work in practice. In the case of a minor-ailments service this will include a detailed explanation of such areas as formulary development, communication and referral systems, protocol development and management of remuneration.
Costings	This is a difficult section to finalise as there may be many hidden costs when setting up a new service. The bid should include a detailed breakdown of all the costs and evidence to support suggested figures. It is useful to liaise with colleagues who have provided a similar service, to ensure that no cost areas have been overlooked. Further information on providing cost information is provided in Chapter 6.
Outcomes expected	The projected number of minor-ailments consultations and the likely outcomes based on similar services should be outlined. This section will include information on potential cost savings of reduced GP appointments on minor ailments and reduced waiting times for an appointment. This will need to be evidence based and linked to the original rationale for the proposed service.
Monitoring, evaluation and clinical governance	The monitoring of the minor-ailments service should include areas such as risk management, complaints procedures and patient satisfaction. An indication of the number and type of audits to be carried out and the identification of training needs will be included in this section.
References	All sections of the bid will need to be fully referenced.

Negotiation skills

Increasingly the pharmacist is required to use negotiation skills when interacting with other healthcare professions and making a business case for a new service. The successful negotiator has well-developed communication skills, is well informed of the needs of all parties involved, and is prepared to be patient in order to obtain their desired outcome. The negotiation process can be described as having four stages: preparation, opening, discussion and closing.[10] The stages of the negotiation process are outlined in Figure 9.3.

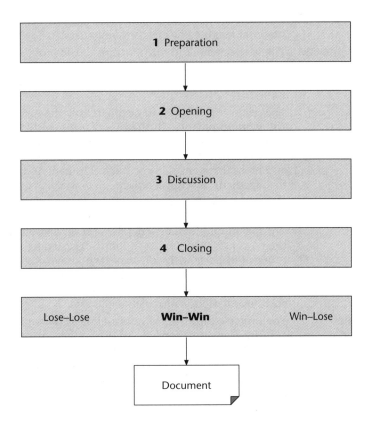

Figure 9.3   Stages of the negotiation process.

Preparation

To prepare for the negotiation, there needs to be a clear understanding of what both parties are aiming to achieve. This will involve collecting and collating factual information in an easily digestible form that can be used as part of the discussion. At this stage a realistic target is set and also the minimum that must be achieved for a satisfactory outcome to the negotiation.

Practical details such as the choice of venue, representatives invited, seating arrangements and timing need to be carefully considered, as these may have a significant bearing on the negotiation process.

Opening

There is a need for order and structure to the opening of the meeting. The opening of the meeting involves listening carefully to the needs of the other side and sharing information. The more information that can be shared, the more trust will be built in the early stages. All opening statements should be friendly and collaborative in tone.

Discussion

The discussion process is where each side elaborates on their specific requirements and seeks clarification where necessary to ensure that there is a clear understanding of the position. It is useful to take notes during a negotiation as this can be a useful way of delaying or hiding the immediate reaction of those involved. These notes will also provide a useful record of what was said, which can later be referred to. Some negotiations can be very complex and it may be necessary to identify areas of potential compromise and concentrate on important areas. A good negotiator is flexible on what they consider to be unimportant matters. It is sometimes useful to accept below the minimum desired outcome on one issue if this can be compensated for in an area that holds more importance. Successful negotiation is not always about winning a case but is an interactive process that involves compromise and agreement. An essential part of discussion is building up good future relationships for future negotiation. For example, if the negotiation is with a local GP practice or PCT about a proposed medicines-management service, mutual respect and trust will be vital for any future collaboration.

Closing

There are three possible outcomes to the close of any negotiation:

- the ideal outcome is a win–win where both sides feel that they have achieved their minimum goals. This outcome is the one that should be aimed for and will prepare the way for future successful negotiation

- the lose–lose outcome is when a stalemate is reached and no party achieves their desired outcome
- the win–lose outcome is when only one party achieves their desired outcome.

Whatever the outcome the agreement should be recorded in writing to avoid any uncertainties at a later date.

Working with hospital pharmacists – discharge schemes

There is a wide variation within hospital pharmacy practice in meeting the medicine-related needs of patients as they are discharged from hospital.[11] Providing seamless pharmaceutical care to patients being discharged from hospital involves proactive multidisciplinary working. In the worst case scenario a patient is delayed and inconvenienced at the point of discharge, because they have to wait for discharge prescriptions to be written and dispensed. Discharge can be further complicated by a lack of communication over changes in medication with the hospital and the GP. An example of a pharmacy-led hospital discharge system is outlined in Example 9.1.

Example 9.1 A hospital discharge scheme

The pharmacy-based scheme at Wrightington Hospital in Wigan has demonstrated beneficial results.[12] The proportion of patients waiting for two hours or more to be discharged was 27% under junior doctors and zero under the pharmacy system. This scheme also demonstrated a reduction in prescription-writing errors and significant cost savings. The procedure adopted consists of the following stages:

- consultant decides that a patient is ready to be discharged
- discharge pharmacist is immediately contacted
- a discharge prescription is written using information from the patient's hospital drug chart, the medication history taken on admission and any special directions from the medical team
- the medicines are dispensed in the normal way, ready for the patient to take home
- the pharmacist counsels the patient or carer about the discharge medication
- the doctor reviews and signs the discharge prescription. This is a much shorter process than writing the discharge prescription

$\rightarrow$

- the prescription form is designed to include space for information for GPs, with explanatory notes on why drug changes have been made and contact details of the discharge service pharmacist
- referral is made to the community liaison pharmacist if the patient requires specific support with medicines after discharge.

As part of a multidisciplinary team the community pharmacist plays a pivotal role in communicating with their hospital colleagues and patient's GP, to ensure that any medication issues are resolved.

Working with specific patient groups

The elderly

There are many opportunities for community pharmacists to become involved in the *National Service Framework for Older People*.[13] Two important milestones that were specified by this NSF are:

- by 2002, all people over 75 years should normally have their medicines reviewed at least annually and those taking four or more medicines should have a 6-monthly review
- by 2004, every PCT will have schemes in place so that older people can get more help from pharmacists in using their medicines.

A resource pack for community pharmacists on this NSF highlights 12 key issues that influence the effectiveness of medication with older people:[14]

- preventable adverse reactions that can lead to hospital admissions
- under-use of medicines such as anti-thrombotic treatment, antidepressants and preventative asthma therapy
- not taking medicines as intended by the prescriber
- inequivalence of repeat prescription quantities leading to wastage
- hospital discharge problems such as a special formulation being prescribed in hospital and no arrangements made for continuity of treatment in the community
- poor two-way communication between hospitals and primary care
- repeat-prescribing issues
- inadequate dosage instructions such as 'take as directed'
- access to pharmacy services for housebound patients or people who have limited mobility
- under-use of carers to support older people in taking their medicine
- detailed medication reviews
- monitoring of patients and potential withdrawal of long-term treatments.

All of these issues will involve pharmacists developing closer links with community-based nurses, local GPs and their support teams.

Coronary heart disease

Coronary heart disease (CHD) is a preventable disease that kills more than 110 000 people in England every year. More than 1.4 million people suffer from angina, and 275 000 people have a heart attack annually. CHD is the biggest killer in the country. The government is committed to reducing the death rate from CHD and stroke and related diseases in people under 75 by at least 40% (to 83.8 deaths per 100 000 population) by 2010.[15]

This NSF outlines 12 National Service standards of care. The standards that are of particular interest to the community pharmacist include:

Standards 1 and 2: reducing heart disease in the population

The NHS and partner agencies should:

- develop, implement and monitor policies that reduce the prevalence of coronary risk factors in the population and reduce inequalities in risks of developing heart disease
- contribute to a reduction in the prevalence of smoking in the local population.

Standards 3 and 4: preventing CHD in high-risk patients

GPs and primary care teams should:

- identify all people with established cardiovascular disease and offer them comprehensive advice and appropriate treatment to reduce their risks
- identify all people at significant risk of cardiovascular disease but who have not developed symptoms, and offer them appropriate advice and treatment to reduce their risks.

All of these standards require a multidisciplinary approach to achieve positive outcomes. There are some excellent examples within community pharmacy practice of involvement in the prevention of CHD. Innovative pharmacy services provide the public with a comprehensive consultation, including blood pressure monitoring, cholesterol testing, body mass index measurement, family history taking and associated lifestyle advice. The result of the pharmacy-based consultation is then transferred directly to the GP in electronic format, to highlight any areas of concern.

Another approach is for the pharmacist to work in partnership with other healthcare professionals and establish drop-in centres in collaboration with local practice nurses, to provide patients with advice on all aspects of coronary care. Table 9.2 outlines potential areas for pharmacist involvement in the *National Service Framework for Coronary Heart Disease*.[15]

Hypertension is a productive area for pharmacists to work with their

Table 9.2 Potential areas for pharmacist involvement in *the National Service Framework for Coronary Heart Disease*[15]

Activity	Examples
Full medication reviews	Identification of medication problems Check that drugs recommended by NSF are in use Identification of concordance issues
Health advice and promotion	Areas of involvement include: smoking, obesity, diet, exercise, alcohol, stress and physical exercise Advice on the symptoms of CHD and other related conditions Establishing smoking-cessation clinics
Health monitoring	Monitoring of cholesterol, blood pressure and glucose levels
Prescribing advice	Advice to local primary care groups and local GPs Advice on NSF guidelines and medicine costs

local medical colleagues as this clinical area is part of the QOF of the GMS contract. The optimum control of hypertension relates to several standards in the *National Service Framework for Older People* as summarised in Table 9.3.[13]

Many people with diabetes also suffer from hypertension and CHD, therefore the *National Service Framework for Diabetes* is also a productive area for pharmacist input as part of a multidisciplinary team.[16]

Diabetes

There are an estimated 2.35 million people with diabetes in England and this is predicted to grow to more than 2.5 million by 2010. The diabetes NSF aims to ensure that people with diabetes, wherever they live, receive the same excellent standard of care.[16] The 'average' community pharmacy serves 156 patients with diabetes.[3]

The *National Service Framework for Diabetes Delivery Strategy* describes how the NHS can achieve the standards of the diabetes NSF.[17] The strategy promotes locally led changes to clinical practice, with an emphasis on systematic care and the integration of primary and secondary care. The

Table 9.3 Control of hypertension and the *National Service Framework for Older People*[13]

NSF standard for older people	Example
Standard five: stroke	Reducing the risk of stroke by maintaining good blood pressure control
Standard six: falls	Regular review and monitoring of antihypertensive medication to prevent falls caused by excessive lowering of blood pressure
Standard eight: the promotion of health and active life in older age	Extension of healthy life expectancy in older people by treating hypertension

strategy recognises the central role of self-management of people with diabetes and states that pharmacists are a regular point of contact for people with diabetes. The pharmacist can become involved in supporting PCTs and GPs to improve the quality of prescribing and inputting into established medicines-management schemes.

As part of the contractual framework, the community pharmacist will offer opportunistic advice on specified public health topics to people with diabetes who present a prescription. This type of advice will also be provided to those at risk of CHD, especially patients with high blood pressure, those who smoke and those who are overweight.

Useful advice for patients with diabetes includes areas such as:

- dietary advice
- blood glucose monitoring to assist people with diabetes to understand their levels better and make appropriate changes to their diet and medication.
- blood pressure and cholesterol checks
- smoking cessation
- advice on alcohol consumption
- medication advice such as offering an MUR service
- signposting footcare problems to a chiropodist
- holiday healthcare to include advice on transport of insulin, timing of medicines to fit in with mealtimes and changes in time zones.

Another area of potential pharmacist involvement is the provision of patient education support groups and programmes. An example of this type of activity is outlined in Example 9.2.

Example 9.2

There are good examples of pharmacist-led diabetes education programmes such as those run by Green Light Pharmacy in London. The pharmacy has two pharmacy-based diabetes support groups to help educate people about their condition, with funding from the health action zone. Both groups meet monthly and a range of topics is covered at each meeting, such as medication, diet and foot care. One group meets in the pharmacy and is for local Bengali men, where there is the facility for measurement of blood pressure, cholesterol and haemoglobin A_{1c} (HbA_{1c}). Dieticians from secondary care or a diabetes nurse are invited in to speak to these meetings. The other group is run for English-speaking patients with diabetes, in partnership with a local charity and meets at the charity's premises.[18]

To meet the needs of people with diabetes there needs to be an integrated approach, which draws on the knowledge and skills of health and social care professionals across a multidisciplinary healthcare team. A useful starting point is for the community pharmacist to make contact with their local diabetes specialist nurse and agree ways of working together.

The way forward

The recent findings of the RPSGB Long-term Conditions project demonstrate convincing evidence of the positive impact that community pharmacy can have in the care of people with asthma, diabetes and coronary heart disease.[3]

There are many opportunities for the proactive community pharmacist to support specific patient groups and establish themselves within the healthcare team. For many years the pharmacist has worked in isolation. A more integrated and open approach to other healthcare professionals is needed to empower individual patients and improve the health of the nation

Implications for practice

Activity 1

Investigate the hospital discharge scheme that is in place in your area. For example telephone the pharmacy department in the local hospital and discuss the scheme with a hospital colleague who has responsibility for the scheme.

- Does the discharge scheme work in practice?
- What are the advantages and disadvantages of the discharge scheme?

Activity 2

Arrange a meeting with a local medical practice to discuss ways of working more closely in a specific clinical area such as hypertension.

- Summarise what your pharmacy could offer in this clinical area.
- Suggest systems of communication between the medical practice and the pharmacy.
- Give examples of the advantages of closer working in this area.

Multiple choice questions

Directions for question 1: each of the questions or incomplete statements in this section is followed by five suggested answers. Select the best answer in each case.

Q1 The 'average' community pharmacy serves approximately the following number of patients with diabetes:

A   20
B   50
C   100
D   150
E   500

Directions for questions 2 and 3: for each numbered question select the one lettered option above it which is most closely related to it. Within each group of questions each lettered option may be used once, more than once, or not at all.

A   Hypertension
B   Diabetes

C   Epilepsy
D   Asthma
E   All of the above

Q2   Which of the above clinical areas are included in the Quality and Outcomes Framework of the GMS contract?

Q3   Which of the above clinical areas relates to several standards in the National Service Framework for Older People?[13]

Directions for questions 4 to 8: each of the questions or incomplete statements in this section is followed by three responses. For each question ONE or MORE of the responses is (are) correct. Decide which of the responses is (are) correct. Then choose:

A   if 1, 2 and 3 are correct
B   if 1 and 2 only are correct
C   if 2 and 3 only are correct
D   if 1 only is correct
E   if 3 only is correct

Directions summarised:
A: 1, 2, 3   B: 1, 2 only   C: 2, 3 only   D: 1 only   E: 3 only

Q4   Aims of the *National Service Framework for Diabetes* include:[16]

1   To enable more people to live free of diabetes
2   To enable more people to live free of the complications of diabetes
3   To reduce inequalities in the quality of care for patients with diabetes

Q5   The *National Service Framework for Diabetes Delivery Strategy* promotes the following:[18]

1   The integration of primary and secondary care
2   Increased hospital-based management of people with diabetes
3   Pharmacist-led diabetes clinics

Q6   Some of the key roles identified in the Department of Health *A Vision for Pharmacy in the New NHS* document is (are):[1]

1   To provide medicines management services, especially for people with short-term conditions
2   To contribute to seamless and safe medicines management throughout the patient journey
3   To support patients as partners in taking medicines

Q7   The aims of the Community Pharmacy Medicines Management Project is (are) to:

1   Develop the partnership between patient, pharmacist and doctor

2   Maximise the skills and training of the community pharmacist
3   Increase collaboration between health professionals in secondary care

Q8   Which of the following areas is (are) recommended for pharmacist involvement with local GPs

1   Advice on medicine costs
2   Advice on NSF guidelines
3   Prescribing advice

Directions for questions 8 to 10: the following questions consist of a statement in the left-hand column followed by a second statement in the right-hand column.
Decide whether the first statement is true or false.
Decide whether the second statement is true or false.
Then choose:

A   if both statements are true and the second statement is a correct explanation of the first statement
B   if both statements are true but the second statement is NOT a correct explanation of the first statement
C   if the first statement is true but the second statement is false
D   if the first statement is false but the second statement is true
E   if both statements are false

Directions summarised:

A:	True	True	second statement is **a correct explanation** of the first
B:	True	True	second statement is **NOT a correct explanation** of the first
C:	True	False	
D:	False	True	
E:	False	False	

Q9

- *Statement 1*: The sharing of patient information between GP and pharmacist and access to a patient's records is permissible when offering a medicines-management service.
- *Statement 2*: The Caldicott Report[8] makes provision for the exchange of information between healthcare professionals in appropriate circumstances.

Q10

- *Statement 1*: A win–win outcome is more desirable than a win–lose outcome in a negotiation.
- *Statement 2*: An important part of the negotiation process is establishing good future relationships with key stakeholders.

Level 1

Clare is a third-year pharmacy undergraduate who is part of an inter-professional group of students. The group includes students of nursing, social work and medicine. The group is asked to look at the case study below and state what specific input their professional group could provide in the overall care package for this patient.

Case study

Mary is 43 years old and has recently been discharged from hospital after an overnight stay following an acute episode of asthma. She lives in a rented two-bedroom flat with her partner and her 12-year-old daughter. The flat is damp and has inadequate heating. Mary has difficulty sleeping and smokes over 30 cigarettes a day. She has tried to give up smoking on several occasions but without success. Her partner is also a smoker and works on the night shift at a local warehouse. Mary works part-time in an accounts office but in the past year has had a lot of absence from work due to various colds and chest infections. An added problem is that Mary has a body mass index (BMI) of 30 and finds it very difficult to exercise due to her asthma. She often feels quite low and sometimes finds it difficult to sleep. Mary feels that she has little support in the home from her partner and daughter.

Her discharge medication from hospital is as follows:

- prednisolone e/c 5 mg tablets 30 mg daily for 5 days
- salbutamol inhaler 2 puffs prn
- beclometasone 200 mcg inhaler 2 puffs bd

- Prepare a summary for Clare to present to her group.
- Suggest possible ways that the different professions represented in the group could work more closely together on this case.

Level 2

Ruth is a preregistration trainee who is working in a community pharmacy in a seaside town that serves a large population of mainly elderly people. Her tutor is the proprietor pharmacist who also employs another pharmacist to look after 34 residential care homes for older people. The pharmacy runs an efficient prescription-collection and delivery service and offers a medicines use review service.

Ruth's tutor explains that she has recently received a letter from the local PCT inviting all local GPs and pharmacists to a meeting to discuss provision of pharmaceutical services for the elderly. The purpose of the meeting is to discuss ways of working more collaboratively to serve the needs of the local elderly population. Ruth's tutor is enthusiastic about this opportunity and suggests that Ruth also attends the meeting.

- Prepare a brief summary for Ruth on how community pharmacists could contribute to the pharmaceutical care of older people.
- Link your summary to the *National Service Framework for Older People*.[13]
- Choose any one area from your summary and outline a brief draft proposal for providing a specific service.

Level 3

Brian is a pharmacist manager of a community pharmacy that supplies medicines to Orchard View, which is a 60-bed residential home. This home represents a considerable amount of Brian's residential home business. In recent months the home has expressed some dissatisfaction with the level of service from his pharmacy and has threatened to change their supplier. Members of the pharmacy team have informed Brian that this home regularly complains about the level of service they receive. The pharmacy team has also commented that this home appears to be very demanding compared to other large homes. Their impression is that the manager of Orchard View is disorganised and does not order the prescriptions in sufficient time for the medication to be prepared. The home seems to constantly be running out of medication. Recently Brian received a letter of complaint from the home manager stating that a member of his staff was abrupt on the telephone when a care worker faxed an interim prescription and the pharmacy claimed that the prescription was illegible.

Brian is very keen to retain this home and arranges a meeting with the home manager.

- Outline the necessary stages involved in Brian's negotiation with this home.
- Suggest possible desired outcomes for Brian in the negotiation with this home.
- For each stage of the negotiation give some indication of the approach he could take.
- Discuss the barriers he may encounter and how these may be overcome.

References

1   Department of Health. *A Vision for Pharmacy in the New NHS*. London: Department of Health, 2003. www.dh.gov.uk/assetRoot/04/06/83/56/ 04068356.pdf (accessed 14 September 2007).

2   All-Party Pharmacy Group. *MPs Launch Inquiry into the Future of Pharmacy*. www.appg.org.uk/Pdf/PharmacyInquirynewsrelease.pdf (accessed 14 September 2007).

3   Royal Pharmaceutical Society of Great Britain. *Long-term Conditions: Integrating community pharmacy – executive summary*. London: Royal Pharmaceutical Society of Great Britain, 2006. www.rpsgb.org.uk/ pdfs/ltcondintegcommphsumm.pdf (accessed 14 September 2007).

4   NHS National Statistics Information Centre. *Prescriptions Dispensed in the Community. Statistics for 1995–2005: England.* www.ic.nhs.uk/webfiles/ publications/prescriptionsdispensed/PrescriptionsDispensed200706_PD F.pdf (accessed 14 September 2007).

5   National Prescribing Centre. *Medicines Management.* www.npc.co.uk/ mms/FiveMinGuides/library/5m_intro_mm.htm (accessed 14 September 2007).

6   Community Pharmacy Medicines Management. www.medicinesman agement.org.uk/ (accessed 14 September 2007).

7   Community Pharmacy Medicines Management. *Resources.* www.medi cinesmanagement.org.uk/resources.php (accessed 14 September 2007).

8   Department of Health. *Report on Review of Patient-identifiable Information* (Caldicott Report). London: Department of Health, 1997. www.dh.gov. uk/en/Publicationsandstatistics/Publications/PublicationsPolicyAndGui dance/DH_4068403 (accessed 14 September 2007).

9   Russell R. How to establish a new community pharmacy service. *Pharm J* 2003; **271**: 237.

10   McGuire R. Negotiation: an important life skill *Pharm J* 2004; **273**: 23–25.

11   Sexton J, Ho YJ, Green CF, Caldwell NA. Ensuring seamless care at hospital discharge: a national survey. *J Clin Pharm Ther* 2000; **25**: 385.

12   Bellingham C. A simple discharge scheme that works. *Pharm J* 2004; **272**: 418.

13   Department of Health. *National Service Framework for Older People*. London: Department of Health, 2001. www.dh.gov.uk/en/Publications andstatistics/Publications/PublicationsPolicyAndGuidance/ DH_4003066 (accessed 18 September 2007).

14   Pharmaceutical Services Negotiating Committee. *National Service Framework for Older People: a guide for community pharmacists*. www.psnc. org.uk/uploaded_txt/NSF_for%20older%20people_Final.pdf (accessed 14 September 2007).

15   Department of Health. *National Service Framework for Coronary Heart Disease*. London: Department of Health, 2000. www.dh.gov.uk/

PublicationsAndStatistics/Publications/PublicationsPolicyAndGuidance /PublicationsPolicyAndGuidanceArticle/fs/en?CONTENT_ID=4094275 &chk=eTacxC (accessed 14 September 2007).

16   Department of Health. *National Service Framework for Diabetes: standards.* London: Department of Health, 2001. www.dh.gov.uk/PublicationsAnd Statistics/Publications/PublicationsPolicyAndGuidance/PublicationsPol icyAndGuidanceArticle/fs/en?CONTENT_ID=4002951&chk=09Kkz1 (accessed 14 September 2007).

17   Department of Health. *National Service Framework for Diabetes Delivery Strategy.* London: Department of Health, 2003. www.dh.gov.uk/en/ Publicationsandstatistics/Publications/PublicationsPolicyAndGuidance/ Browsable/DH_4097539 (accessed 14 September 2007).

18   News item. Pharmacists need to be proactive in the care of patients with diabetes. *Pharm J* 2003; **270**: 75–76. www.pharmj.com/Editorial/ 20030118/news/news_diabetes.html (accessed 14 September 2007).

Answers

Chapter	1	2	3	4	5	6	7	8	9
Q1	C	B	B	C	C	B	B	B	D
Q2	D	C	B	A	D	B	B	D	E
Q3	E	D	A	B	E	D	D	B	A
Q4	D	C	A	A	B	A	A	A	A
Q5	D	B	E	B	A	C	B	C	D
Q6	A	A	D	A	D	D	B	B	C
Q7	C	E	B	C	E	C	A	E	B
Q8	A	A	B	C	A	C	A	A	A
Q9	D	A	A	A	A	A	D	D	A
Q10	A	A	D	D	A	B	A	A	A

Case studies

Chapter 1

Level 1

Write four objectives for John to include in his portfolio that could be achievable over the next year.

- Reference to SMART objective writing
- Areas of development that need to be considered include:
  - gaining practical pharmacy experience
  - finding out more information about hospital pharmacy
  - communication and team-working skills
  - presentation skills.

Example objective

To speak to a minimum of two hospital pharmacists and arrange to visit a local hospital pharmacy department, or attend an open day.

Level 2

Using SMART objectives outline a personal development plan for John *before* he starts work as a community pharmacist in his first pharmacy.

Personal and professional development needs would include areas such as:

- development of communication skills and effective team working
- areas specific to community pharmacy such as responding to symptoms
- management skills required to work with a small team
- awareness of the community pharmacy contract.

These would need to be written as SMART objectives.

Level 3: advisory service to care homes

Outline the reflection section of John's CPD entry.

- I want to learn about offering an advisory service to residential care homes.
- This learning objective has been identified in response to an informal meeting with my line manager and a discussion on developing the pharmacy business.
- This objective is driven by my employer.
- I need knowledge on current good practice on medicines management in care homes and also improved communication skills to work with care home staff.
- Link to specific competencies (select from general competences for pharmacists and also specific competences for pharmacists working in community practice).

Outline the planning section of John's CPD entry.

- Learning objective has been allocated three months to achieve.
- Impact on myself (high).
- Impact on service users (high).
- Impact on colleagues (low).
- Impact on organisation (high).
- (1) Shadow pharmacist colleague who offers this service. Advantage is that there will be the opportunity to ask questions and clarify information and procedures. Disadvantage is that it will be time consuming.
- (2) Complete CPPE training package on care homes – mandatory requirement.

- (3) Attend two training evenings provided by primary care trust.
- (2) and (3) are mandatory requirements in order to be accredited to be able to offer this service. (1) needs careful planning but would be a useful way of building confidence in this area.

Chapter 2

Level 1

> What advice would you give to Sheetal to ensure that the next meeting runs more smoothly and is more productive?

This case study is based on effective meetings management of a diverse group of students. To maximise the time spent at the next meeting Sheetal should consider the following:

- preparation for the meeting should include communication with all group members and the allocation of a chairperson and scribe. These roles should be rotated in future meetings
- a purpose for the meeting and a timed agenda should be agreed in advance and circulated
- the role of the chairperson should be agreed by the group and specific ground rules discussed and documented before the meeting commences. The importance of including all group members and not allowing one person to monopolise the meeting should be emphasised
- after the meeting the scribe should circulate meeting notes, including action points. All action points should be monitored, and preparations made for the next meeting.

Level 2

> Produce a brief bullet-pointed list of constructive advice for Michelle on how she should plan a meeting.

- The purpose of the meeting should be clearly stated.
- Decide who should be invited to the meeting.
- Set date, time and venue.
- Provide some background information or possible options for the event and invite suggestions prior to the meeting with a deadline for a reply.
- Check and collate responses.
- Produce and circulate an agenda.

> Produce a brief bullet-pointed list of constructive advice for Michelle on a suitable agenda for this meeting with proposed timing.

The agenda needs to include an introduction to the purpose of the meeting and a structured discussion of each suggested health-promotion activity. Each section of the agenda should have an allocated time to ensure that the discussion is focused. The meeting should include a summary of all agreed activities. There should be a space for any other business, the content of which should be agreed at the start of the meeting.

> Produce a brief bullet-pointed list of constructive advice for Michelle on how she should follow up the meeting.

Notes of the meeting should be summarised, including responsibility for any action points and the timeframe for each action point noted. This should be circulated as soon as possible after the meeting. Michelle should monitor each action point and check that all allocated tasks are completed within the agreed timeframe. Details of any future meeting should also be circulated.

Level 3

> Carry out a SWOT analysis of this business

(S) Strengths

- Good access and parking facilities
- Some loyal customers
- No direct competition

(W) Weaknesses

- Very low turnover of both NHS and counter sales
- Large amount of stock
- Staff poorly motivated
- Neglected business and poor management history

(O) Opportunities

- Development of prescription-collection service
- Large floor area for potential future development of business

(T) Threats

- Main threat is lack of central location and neglect of business

> What are John's priorities as a new manager? Construct a time chart of suggested actions for John during his first 2 months as a manager.

Month 1

Week 1

- Set up a business plan with key performance indicators and meet with all staff to communicate priorities for business.
- Set up meetings with all local medical practices and launch prescription-collection and delivery service.

Week 2

- Carry out a training needs analysis for the staff, matched to the business plan.
- Meet with all staff to discuss individual training needs to include dispensary working.
- Introduce performance management process for staff.
- Set up appropriate training programme for all staff.

Week 3

- Set up a programme of dispensary stock reduction, major cleaning and dispensary reorganisation.
- Review all dispensary SOPs and check staff competence in main areas.

Week 4

- Make decision on use of retail area and ensure full-time supervisor takes full responsibility for sales area. This will involve checking sales data and remerchandising.

Month 2

- Review all of the key performance indicators and monitor progress. Hold a review meeting with all staff members.

Chapter 3

Level 1

Make a list of criteria that you would suggest for inclusion in a marking scheme for presentation.

Some suggested criteria for the assessment of presentation skills could include areas such as:

- clear statement of presentation aim and objectives
- person presenting is audible and clear
- appropriate personal demeanour (eye contact, confidence etc)
- accuracy of presentation content
- content pitched at an appropriate level

- presentation is well structured and fluid
- presentation is summarised
- questions are handled confidently and accurately
- visual aids are clear and support the presentation.

Level 2

> Kerry is asked to produce an outline plan of a 30-minute training session on this product area.

Suggested ideas for a training session on sale of cough medicines:

- brainstorm – common questions on cough medicines (3 minutes)
- define objectives of training session (5 minutes)
- types of cough (3 minutes)
- warning signs – referral (3 minutes)
- case study – group activity (5 minutes)
- role-play activity (5 minutes)
- quick quiz (3 minutes)
- check objectives and set future personal objectives (3 minutes).

> What specific preregistration performance standards relate to this activity?

Preregistration performance standards that relate to this activity can be selected from the areas B1 (communicate effectively) and B2 (work effectively with others).

Level 3

> Marie has been asked by her area manager to produce a proposed training plan for this pharmacy, what should she include?

The main priorities for Marie could include the following:

- introduce a training timetable into the working week where protected training time is allocated to all staff members
- introduce a formal mentoring system
- introduction of a CPD process for Jeanne and Sandy
- if possible move individual staff to work in other pharmacies within the multiple for short periods of time to develop specific skills
- within the pharmacy it may be useful to move Sandy (pharmacy technician) to the dispensary to supervise Sharon.
- Jeanne could be moved away from the main dispensary to service the residential care homes.
- Dan should be introduced to dispensing duties and be supervised by Sandy
- the newly appointed trainee dispenser could be split between Sandy and Jeanne
- Marie would need to offer regular coaching to Lorna and Beth to improve performance on the medicine counter.

Chapter 4

Level 1

Prepare a brief summary for Tamara, using bullet points, of how the contractual framework for community pharmacy can relate to GPs, nurses and social workers.

GPs and nurses

- Link of essential services such as repeat dispensing, public health, signposting and self-care to working with GPs
- Impact on time spent by GPs on minor ailments
- Interaction with GPs and practice nurses in the delivery of an MUR service
- Link of specific enhanced services such as smoking-cessation and minor-ailments schemes.

Social workers

- Impact of repeat dispensing service on patients and carers
- Potential impact of MUR service on hospital admissions
- Additional support under the DDA
- More co-ordinated referral process
- Possibility of innovative enhanced services where pharmacy and social services work more closely together, e.g. domiciliary visiting schemes.

Level 2

What issues are involved in this case?

- Requirements that apply to pharmacy services under the DDA such as making reasonable adjustments including the provision of extra help or changing the way that services are provided.
- Dispensary team appears to ignore customer query and there is no protocol in place.

What could Ryan have done differently?

- Ryan is very inexperienced and was relying on support from the pharmacy team in the absence of his tutor.
- Ideally he should have made an appointment for the customer to have had a consultation with the pharmacist to have her needs properly assessed. As Ryan is only in the first few weeks of training he would be unlikely to have come across this problem.
- By trying to take initiative he made the wrong decision (possibly under pressure). He should have taken the patient's contact details so that a more detailed conversation could take place.

What preregistration performance standards could this incident relate to?

■ The most relevant performance standard to this scenario is A1.3: Recognise your personal and professional limitations and refer appropriately.

Level 3

Identify the clinical governance issues in this case study.

■ Lack of formal induction for a new member of staff
■ No evidence of referral to SOPs or new member of staff assessed as competent
■ New member of staff not appropriately briefed, lack of support and absence of a mentoring process
■ Inappropriate initial tasks allocated that involve direct contact with members of the public
■ Incidents from the diary indicate the seriousness of handing out the wrong prescription item without an adequate identity check and lone working of an untrained person on the medicine counter.

Chapter 5

Level 1

Using bullet points summarise the issues that need to be highlighted with this patient and their GP.

■ Discuss BMI and lifestyle management.
■ To control pain, the paracetamol should be taken as a regular dose rather than a prn dose.
■ Eliminate the co-codamol tablets.
■ Explore cough and check it is not a side-effect of ACE inhibitor.
■ Discuss the purpose of each medicine and the importance of taking regularly.
■ Discuss ways of improving compliance.

Level 2

What areas would you need to explore before making your final action plan?

Areas that would need to be considered would include:

■ inhaler technique and compliance
■ use of a spacer to assist patient with inhaler usage
■ smoking cessation advice
■ the dose of Slo-Phyllin and possible adjustment as the smoking has reduced

- known side-effects – for example the palpitations – possibly due to salbutamol
- lifestyle advice – exercise and weight control.

Level 3

What suggestions would you offer to Bill to increase the level of uptake of MURs in his pharmacy?

- Need to explore reasons behind Bill's reluctance to become involved in this service
- Discussion with local GPs on the advantages of this service and how the results will be communicated
- Use of appropriate publicity
- Targeting of specific patient groups in line with local priorities
- Training of the pharmacy team to identify suitable patients and discuss the service with potential patients.

Chapter 6

Level 1

What areas of discussion do you think Lucy's tutor should include in the first meeting with this client?

- A full history should be documented
- Detailed discussion on client AB's motivation to stop smoking
- Talking through a typical day of smoking – identification of high-risk situations
- Emphasis on the benefits of stopping smoking
- Talk about coping strategies for stressful situations and dealing with cravings
- Reinforce positive lifestyle change to increase weight loss
- Set a quit date – provision of any useful supportive material
- Explanation of NRT
- Selection of NRT product – gum would be suitable as AB is a behaviourally dependent smoker
- Explanation of use of gum and dosage and provision of 2 weeks' supply for use after the quit date
- Make an appointment for 2 weeks after the quit date and offer intermediate telephone support.

Level 2

Nick is asked by his tutor to look at the PMR record for Mrs Rose and prepare a suitable answer that they can discuss together before the tutor returns the phone call. What would you advise Nick to include in his response?

- Use liquid formulations (if available) if resident is unable to swallow tablets
- From the PMR:
  - co-codamol 8/500 effervescent tablets
  - senna available as Senokot syrup
  - amoxicillin available as 250 mg/5 ml oral suspension
- Specials manufacturing of other liquid formulations such as levothyroxine – cost implication/short shelf-life
- Discuss legal implications of crushing solid-dose forms and the importance of agreement from all parties and signed documentation.

Level 3

What specific points do you think Meera should include in her presentation to address the concerns of her colleagues?

- Emphasis on training of all staff involved, the use of standard operating procedures and clear quality indicators
- Participation in annual PCO audit of service provision
- Piloting of service to fit in with local needs and ways of working
- Piloting of electronic closed loop communication systems to avoid excessive paperwork and duplication of effort.

Chapter 7

Level 1

How do you think the pharmacist should respond to this patient?

The pharmacist's response should communicate the following:

- positive benefits of maintaining PMRs such as being able to check individual medication, dose changes and interactions
- the NHS contractual obligation when offering a dispensing service to keep records, in order to be able to offer a safe and effective service
- reassure the patient that all records are subject to data-protection legislation, and outline how the data are maintained securely
- explain that Carla is working in line with standard procedures to ensure that data are accurate and up to date.

Level 2

After hearing Neil's version of events, Neil's tutor asked him what he would have done differently. How should the locum pharmacist have responded to the situation?

The pharmacist should have:

- listened carefully to Mr Jones and allowed him to make his complaint fully
- quickly retrieved the original prescription from the file
- dispensed the correct item using the original prescription
- offered an apology to Mr Jones and assured him that a full investigation will be made into the error
- asked Mr Jones if the incorrect item could be retained in the pharmacy, and stored this item securely and separately from other dispensing stock
- made a full record of the incident and informed the superintendent pharmacist or their representative
- investigated the root cause of the error and involved other members of the pharmacy team in this process.

Level 3

What suggestions would you give to the proprietor of this business?

Areas for Mike to consider include:

- the size of the dispensary area in relation to the retail floor area
- a consultation room that is future-proof
- a separate dispensing area for the residential homes that is connected to the main dispensary to facilitate supervision
- a large area for the repeat-prescription service and adequate storage for these items
- the workflow of the dispensary and position of PMR systems
- the use of space and adequate space for all pharmacy services such as waste disposal
- ease of access and consideration of mainly elderly customers
- a suitable consultation area for possible use by other healthcare professions
- an area for health-promotion displays.

Chapter 8

Level 1

How do you recognise the clinical features of athlete's foot?

- Most prevalent in adolescents and young adults
- Infection in the toe webs, especially the fourth web space (next to the little toe)
- Skin appears white and soggy
- Itchy and feet have a tendency to smell
- Dermatophytic fungi prefer moist conditions – feet damp after sports and probably not dried thoroughly
- All of the above features evident in the case study
- Sometimes the infection spreads to the sole and instep of the foot and in persistent cases the nail may become involved (becomes dull, opaque and

yellow – brittle and crumbling); the nail is more likely to be involved in older adults

What questions would you ask Mark Dean to ensure that his condition does not require referral?

Referral is needed if:

- there is involvement of the nail as described above – refer as possible systemic treatment needed
- OTC treatment has failed
- there is any suspected facial or scalp involvement.

Critically discuss the availability of OTC products for athlete's foot and make an evidence-based recommendation for this patient.

- Undecenoates: Mycota, Monphytol – positive reports of efficacy from Cochrane review
- Tolnaftate: Mycil – limited trial data
- Imidazoles: clotrimazole (Canesten, Canesten AF), ketoconazole (Daktarin Gold) greater efficacy than above two groups – no clinically significant differences in cure rates between different imidazoles
- Allyamines: terbinafine (Lamisil AT) – allyamines shown to be more efficacious than imidazoles in comparative trials

Level 2

What are the benchmark standards that Yunus could select when designing this audit?

Benchmark standards could include:

- customer is given clear dosage instructions including the maximum dosage in 24 hours
- customer is warned about not taking additional products that contain paracetamol.

How could the audit be designed?

- Yunus would need to work in close proximity to the medicines counter and observe all staff when they either recommend or are asked specifically for paracetamol-based products. Yunus would need to ensure that the audit takes place over a defined time period and covers all staff members involved in the sale of medicines.

What are some of the practical problems and limitations of this type of audit?

- Staff may behave differently when being observed and this may distort data.

- Yunus may find it difficult to carry out audit and it will be very time consuming.
- Customers may find the audit intrusive.

Level 3

Highlight Colin's concerns about this incident

- Colin's concerns relate to the quality of advice given in relation to colic and weaning. Advice given is anecdotal rather than in line with Department of Health recommendations.
- This is well below the standard expected when a member of the public seeks specific advice in a pharmacy.

How should Colin approach Laura with these concerns?

- To manage this type of behaviour Colin will need to speak to Laura privately off the shop floor and ensure that the conversation is uninterrupted.
- Ideally this should be done as part of a performance review.
- The positive aspects of Laura's work should be emphasised.
- The importance of evidence-based recommendations and national guidelines rather than personal opinion should be discussed.
- This could be approached in a generic way by giving specific examples using other product areas.

Chapter 9

Level 1

Prepare a summary for Clare to present to her group

Pharmacist input could include:

- demonstration of inhaler usage and counselling on medication
- smoking-cessation advice and support
- weight-management advice and support
- signposting to other healthcare and social agencies that could offer support.

Suggest possible ways that the different professions represented in the group could work more closely together on this case.

Closer working could include:

- participation in a hospital discharge scheme to improve communication between secondary and primary care
- communication with the social worker to resolve accommodation problems that will impact on health
- closer working with the GP and nurse.

Level 2

> Prepare a brief summary for Ruth on how community pharmacists could contribute to the pharmaceutical care of older people

■ Ruth's summary should include some of the issues that influence the effectiveness of medication with older people. (see: Working with specific patient groups, p. 247).

> Link your summary to the *National Service Framework for Older People.*

■ Discuss important milestones in NSF such as regular medication reviews and enabling older people to get more out of their medicines.

> Choose any one area from your summary and outline a brief draft proposal for providing a specific service.

■ Examples of service areas that could be developed include hospital discharge schemes and domiciliary visiting.

Level 3

> Outline the necessary stages involved in Brian's negotiation with this home.
>
> Suggest possible outcomes for Brian in the negotiation with this home.
>
> For each stage of the negotiation give some indication of the approach he could take.
>
> Discuss the barriers he may encounter and how these may be overcome.

Negotiation will involve the following stages:

■ *preparation*: before the meeting Brian needs to consider what both parties are aiming to achieve and set a realistic minimum target of what he needs from the meeting. The meeting time needs to be set and it is important that the key people involved are all invited to the meeting
■ *opening*: this stage will involve listening to the viewpoint of the residential home and finding out what they are trying to achieve
■ *discussion*: at this stage both sides will need to elaborate on their requirements and give specific details. For Brian this will involve details of a service level agreement that covers areas such as the time needed to dispense medication into a monitored dose system and procedures for telephoned or faxed prescriptions
■ *closing*: a record is made of the agreed outcome.

Barriers encountered may involve a difference in opinion over the level of service required. Brian will need to emphasise that an efficient service will need clear guidelines in order to operate effectively. The importance of patient safety and clinical governance will need to be clearly communicated.

Appendix 1

Example of a medicines use review form

At the time of going to press a new version of the medicines use review form was introduced. The new simplified format aims to provide a more accessible overview for the GP. The new form can be downloaded from the PSNC website. The original version of the form can continue to be used until the end of September 2008.

Community Pharmacy Medicines Use Review & Prescription Intervention Service

Patient Details				
Date of review: 01/05/07	**Title:** Mrs	**Name:** AB		**NHS Patient Code:**
				Pharmacy (PMR) ID:
Address: 4 The High Street Newtown				**DOB:** 02/01/41
				Tel:
GP: Dr RS		**GP address:** Central Medical Practice Newtown		

Recording of patient's informed consent (must be completed before the review can proceed)

Patient has received information on and consented to the review process.	☒
Patient has agreed that information may be shared with their GP.	☒
Patient has agreed that information may be shared with others such as carers.	☐
Specify others by name:	

Reason for review:		Pharmacist identified	☒	or
Annual Review (MUR)	☒	Referral from	☐	
Prescription Intervention	☐			

What would the patient like to get out of the review? (including the need for information)
To find out more information about medication

Basic health data

Significant previous ADRs: None	Known allergies/sensitivities: None
Medical history as described by patient and from information recorded in PMR	Monitoring as described by patient and from information recorded in PMR
Angina	**Not using any GTN - experienced headaches when used this in the past**
Hypertension	BP - not known, but has regular check up
Primary hypercholesterolaemia	TC = 4.9
Type II diabetes (controlled by diet)	regular blood glucose monitoring

Name of pharmacist conducting the review:	
Pharmacy name & address:	

Location of review:	**Outcome of review:**
Pharmacy ☒	
Other location ☐	Copy of care plan given to patient ☒
	Referral made to GP ☐
(state location used)	Pharmacist actions completed and
Telephone ☐	recorded in care plan ☒
(record reason why face to face was not possible)	

(Final version)

Patient Name: **DOB:**

Prescribed medicine and dosage regimen	Dosage regimen as patient takes it (including OTC & complementary therapies)	Patient's knowledge of the medicine's use	Compliance			
			always	*frequent*	*seldom*	*never*
1. Aspirin 75 mg	One in the morning	To thin the blood	☐	☒	☐	☐
2. Atenolol 25 mg	One in the morning	Blood pressure	☐	☒	☐	☐
3. Lisinopril 20 mg	One in the morning	Blood pressure	☐	☒	☐	☐
4. Glyceryl trinitrate tablets 500 mcg	1–2 under the tongue repeated as required	Angina	☐	☐	☐	☒
5. Simvastatin 40 mg	One at night	Cholesterol	☒	☐	☐	☐
6. Paracetamol 500 mg tablets	2 every 4 hours if required	Joint pain	☒	☐	☐	☐
7. Codeine phosphate 30 mg	one or two four times a day	Joint pain	☒	☐	☐	☐
8.			☐	☐	☐	☐
9.			☐	☐	☐	☐
10.			☐	☐	☐	☐
11.			☐	☐	☐	☐
12.			☐	☐	☐	☐
13.			☐	☐	☐	☐
14.			☐	☐	☐	☐

Explanatory notes:

Patient's knowledge of the medicine's use – record what the patient thinks the medicine is for and highlight where response would indicate need for further information.

Compliance – Use open, non-judgemental questions to establish how the medicine is being taken, and tick the box which best indicates the patient's level of compliance, i.e. always takes the medicines as prescribed through to never takes the medicine as prescribed. Leave blank for 'PRN' medicines.

Patient Name: **DOB:**

Is the formulation appropriate?		Is the medicine working?			Are side effects present?		General comments
yes	no	yes	no	unknown	yes	no	
1. ☒	☐	☒	☐	☐	☐	☒	Take with or after food. Low-dose aspirin for primary prevention of coronary events, when BP is controlled
2. ☒	☐	☒	☐	☐	☐	☒	Long duration of action and must only be taken once daily. It is important not to stop taking this without advice
3. ☒	☐	☒	☐	☐	☐	☒	Works by relaxing and widening blood vessels to reduce BP
4. ☒	☐	☐	☐	☒	☒	☐	Helps stop angina pain. To be taken immediately before any exertion that is known to cause pain. Tablets must be discarded after 8 weeks of opening
5. ☒	☐	☒	☐	☐	☐	☒	Importance of taking at night for maximum effectiveness. Report any unexplained muscle pain, tenderness or weakness immediately
6. ☒	☐	☒	☐	☐	☐	☒	Care with other OTC products – check to see if they contain paracetamol
7. ☒	☐	☒	☐	☐	☒	☐	Side-effect of constipation evident
8. ☐	☐	☐	☐	☐	☐	☐	
9. ☐	☐	☐	☐	☐	☐	☐	
10. ☐	☐	☐	☐	☐	☐	☐	
11. ☐	☐	☐	☐	☐	☐	☐	
12. ☐	☐	☐	☐	☐	☐	☐	
13. ☐	☐	☐	☐	☐	☐	☐	
14. ☐	☐	☐	☐	☐	☐	☐	

Explanatory notes:

Is the formulation appropriate? – use to identify problems with formulation, e.g. swallowing difficulties suggest a liquid product may be more suitable, include poor technique with inhaler devices here.

Is the medicine working? – if you have objective evidence such as BP or cholesterol level then you may indicate whether the medicine is effective or not. In many cases this may be a subjective response based on the patient's view of their treatment. In other cases it may be unknown such as antiplatelet therapy.

Are side-effects present? – indicate patients reported response supplemented by a professional decision as to which drug a particular side-effect may be attributable to.

General comments – add any additional information here for example if you have ticked a positive response for side-effects present it would be helpful to add detail (such as cough and skin rash) which may help you when you develop your action plan and when completing a follow-up review with the same patient at a later date.

Medicines Use Review Action Plan

		Date of review:	01/05/07
Patient's name:	Mrs AB		
		Date of Birth:	02/01/41
		NHS Patient Code:	
		GP's name:	Dr RS

Medicines Use Issue	Priority	Proposed Action	Action by	Outcome if known with dates
Diabetes	Med	Advised Mrs AB re diet, regular meals, reduction in fat, 5 portions of fruit and veg a day and reduce alcohol intake	Mrs AB	
Hypertension	Med	Lifestyle factors may influence BP and risk of developing heart disease/stroke. Discussed weight reduction, regular exercise	Mrs AB	
Pain	High	Pain relief needs to reviewed as evidence of over use of codeine for joint pain. Consider prescribing laxative for constipation	Dr RS	

Pharmacist name (block capitals)	RPSGB registration number	Pharmacist signature	Telephone number of pharmacist:

Next steps:

☐ **PATIENT:**
This is your copy; please retain it for your personal use. You may wish to show it to other healthcare professionals if you wish to share this information.

☒ Please make an appointment with your GP to discuss within

☐ 2 ☐ weeks.

☐ Take this form to your next scheduled GP appointment.

☒ Follow your actions agreed above.

☐ **GENERAL PRACTITIONER:**
This is your copy; please retain a copy in your patient's notes.

☐ For information only – no action required.

☒ Please review the actions proposed above.

This review is based on information available to the pharmacist held on the pharmacy medication records and from information provided by the patient.

Index

Page numbers in *italics* refer to figures or tables